PRIMARY CARE OF HAND INJURIES

'Tis God gives skill,
But not without men's hands: He could not make
Antonio Stradivari's violins
without Antonio.

GEORGE ELIOT
IN STRADIVARIUS

Primary Care of Hand Injuries

William L. Newmeyer, M.D.

Assistant Clinical Professor of Surgery
University of California
San Francisco, California

LEA & FEBIGER / 1979 / PHILADELPHIA

Library of Congress Cataloging in Publication Data

Newmeyer, William L
    Primary care of hand injuries.

    Bibliography: p.
    Includes index.
    1. Hand—Wounds and injuries. I. Title.
[DNLM: 1. Hand injuries—Therapy. 2. Hand in-
juries—Surgery. WE830 M556p]
RD559.N48   617'.1   78-31444
ISBN 0-8121-0669-5

Published in Great Britain by Henry Kimpton Publishers, London
Printed in the United States of America

Print Number   3   2   1

Dedicated with love to my wife

NANCY

*who probably did not know what she was in for in 1962
and to our children*

Carla (1967)
and
Thomas (1970)

*who had no choice, their forbearance and support
made it all possible.*

Preface

INJURIES to the hand are among the most frequent accidents to occur in both home and industry. About 25% of all emergency department visits are made for treatment of hand problems, and 30% to 40% of all industrial accidents are hand injuries. Although these injuries are rarely life-threatening, they often jeopardize the patient's livelihood and may cause considerable misery. Perhaps with no other part of the body does the final therapeutic result depend so heavily upon the quality of primary care.

With the encouraging growth in the primary care specialities of emergency medicine and family practice, the quality of primary care of the hand has improved. Since 1974 a course on primary care of the injured hand has been given to a number of groups—mainly emergency physicians—around the country. The response has been enthusiastic, and this book is based upon the format that evolved from this course. Thus, this text is written for physicians whose main interest is primary care, in the hope that their application of the principles discussed and their experience in the techniques described here will reduce the length of disability and improve the final function for all persons with hand injuries. Residents in surgical specialties will also find this book useful. This text is not directed to surgeons who deal definitively with hand problems, although I welcome the scrutiny of the content and the observations of my colleagues in hand surgery.

Most of the techniques and procedures presented here can be carried out in a well-equipped outpatient facility. Almost all of the materials and techniques that I have recommended I have also used extensively. In many instances, other materials or methods may achieve a similar outcome; those that I have described have been proven successful in clinical practice when the principles of their application have been faithfully followed. This is not an encyclopedic treatise, but a personal statement on how primary hand care can be done successfully. Readers are encouraged to expand their knowledge of care of the hand through further education, and to modify and improve the techniques presented here after they have mastered the basics. Indeed, I would like to know about such modifications and improvements.

No primary care physician is encouraged to carry out procedures with which he or she does not feel comfortable. In large metropolitan areas, some problems are better referred to specialists, for legal reasons if for none other. By the same token, there is no reason to send a patient several hundred miles to undergo a procedure that might easily be accomplished in 45 or 60 minutes.

The book is divided into two parts. Part I is devoted to a discussion of basic elements common to all hand injuries and necessary for the treatment of all hand injuries; in Part II these principles are applied to the treatment of specific problems. Basic to all hand care is a knowledge of functional anatomy, which is discussed in Chapter 1. This anatomic knowledge is applied in Chapter 2, Diagnosis and Referral of Hand Injuries and Afflictions, in which a method of history-taking and examination is outlined to help the physician arrive at a rapid, correct diagnosis and formulate a plan of treatment. The next three chapters emphasize the "nuts and bolts" of emergency hand care: materials and techniques essential to proper examination of the hand (Chapter 3); dressing and splinting the injured hand (Chapter 4); and anesthesia, incisions, and antibiotics useful in primary hand care (Chapter 5). Part I concludes with a statement on the vital need of the patient to understand and assume responsibility for his role in the management and rehabilitation of hand problems.

The second part of the book considers the application of these principles to specific problems. The correct treatment of these problems depends absolutely on adherence to the techniques outlined in Part I. The specific problems considered include those that can be treated definitively by the primary care physician, those that require referral for hospitalization or the attention of a specialist, and those that may be managed by either approach depending upon the circumstances.

Inevitably, some will find the information too detailed and others will find it too sparse. No doubt, some aspects have been omitted unintentionally. Hopefully, what is here will prove useful to the reader and beneficial to the patient.

WILLIAM L. NEWMEYER

San Francisco, California

Acknowledgments

MANY people aided me directly and indirectly in conceptualizing, writing, and producing this book. I thank Helen Caldwell and Kitty McKnew who typed and retyped the various drafts. Kelly Ann Alsedek turned my rough sketches into finished line drawings and I am indebted to her for this. I am grateful to the staff at Lea & Febiger for advice and guidance in the preparation of this book.

I want to thank my parents publicly for their support and encouragement over the years. I thank J. William Littler, M. D., and Richard G. Eaton, M. D. for advice given over many years and especially for my early training in hand surgery.

Colleagues in the field of emergency medicine who were most helpful are Karl Mangold, M. D., and John McCabe, M. D. William P. Graham, III, M. D., has been helpful to me in medical writing.

My office nurse, Janet Carlson, R.N., has helped in the preparation of this book in many ways and I thank her for this help.

Residents, fellows, and practicing physicians who have helped by providing photographs and critically reading various chapters include: Harold McDonald, M. D., Morton R. Maser, M. D., Wallace Jones, M. D., John Weeter, M. D., Harrison Smith, M. D., Michael Casey, M. D., Richard Leonards, M. D., and Alan Johnson, M. D. My sincere thanks go to all of them.

Hundreds of patients have helped me gain greater insight into problems of the hand and I hope this volume will lessen the misery and disability of people with hand problems in the future.

My greatest thanks and appreciation go to my colleague in the practice of hand surgery, Eugene S. Kilgore, Jr., M. D. He has given me both the opportunity to see large numbers of patients with hand problems and the benefit of his enormous practical wisdom about the hand distilled from vast experience and an always enquiring mind.

W. L. N.

Contents

PART ONE

Basic Elements of Hand Care

It is better to light one candle than curse the darkness.

MOTTO OF THE CHRISTOPHER SOCIETY

1

Functional Anatomy of the Hand

P RIMARY care of hand injuries requires a good working knowledge of the surface topography of the hand, the structures beneath the surface landmarks, and the interdependence of these underlying structures on one another. This chapter elucidates these relationships. Readers are encouraged to supplement this material by referring to the references cited at the end of the chapter.

Topography and Terminology of the Hand

The use of precise terminology in describing and recording hand injuries is important. The hand and digits have a dorsal surface and a volar (or palmar) surface. They have a radial (thumb) side and an ulnar (little finger) side (Fig. 1-1). The terms medial and lateral are confusing if applied to the hand. In the hand, lateral is used to refer to structures on either side of the digits, such as the radial lateral or ulnar lateral band. The term medial is not used.

The prominent soft tissue protuberances on the proximal palm are referred to as the thenar wad (on the radial side at the base of the thumb) and the hypothenar wad (on the ulnar side at the base of the little finger). Most palms have one predominant crease, the midpalmar crease, and two less prominent creases, the proximal and distal creases.

3

Fingers are named thumb, index, long (or middle), ring, and little. Digits (or rays) are numbered I, II, III, IV, and V (Fig. 1-2). Numbering fingers, as is often done, may cause confusion, because the fourth finger may be regarded by some to be the little finger, and by others, the ring finger.

The thumb has two phalanges and the other digits have three each. It is convenient to refer to proximal and distal phalanges of the thumb and to proximal, middle, and distal phalanges of each of the other digits. Each digit has a metacarpophalangeal (MCP) joint. The first carpometacarpal (CM) joint is referred to as the basal joint of the thumb. The thumb has a single interphalangeal (IP) joint; each of the other digits has a proximal interphalangeal (PIP) joint and a distal interphalangeal (DIP) joint. These abbreviations for joints are used in the remainder of the text (Fig. 1-3).

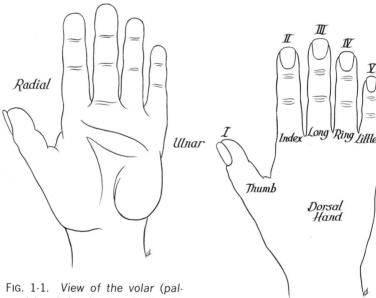

FIG. 1-1.   View of the volar (palmar) hand showing terminology to be used in describing borders of the hand or digits. The other side of the hand is the dorsal side.

FIG. 1-2.   Number the digits and name the fingers to avoid confusion in terminology.

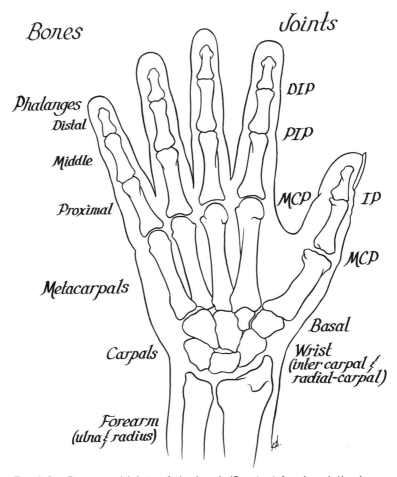

FIG. 1-3. *Bones and joints of the hand. (See text for description.)*

The Skin and Nails

The skin of the hand is highly specialized to permit maximal mobility, sensibility, and adaptability. The volar skin and the dorsal skin are quite different. The volar skin is thick and tethered to firm underlying fascia with maximal fixation at the palmar and joint creases (Fig. 1-4). It is highly sensible. The thickness of the skin makes it less susceptible to burns, abrasions, and other injuries than the dorsal skin. The underlying fascia holds the skin firmly, preventing sliding and slipping over the underlying soft tissue and skeletal structures when objects are grasped. Loss of this fixation, especially in fingerpads, can seriously impair hand function. Sensibility on palmar surfaces, particularly on the finger-pads, is acute, with two-point discrimination at about 4 mm. Along with this acute sensibility is a remarkable toughness that allows a two-digit pinch up to 8 kg. and a hand grasp to 60 or more kg.

The soft tissue structures beneath the volar skin are well protected and include the flexor tendons, the major sensory and intrinsic motor nerves, and the principal portion of the arterial blood supply.

The dorsal skin, by contrast, is thin and loosely attached to the underlying dorsal hand structures. Combined with the intrinsic elasticity of the skin, this looseness allows the stretch required for normal finger flexion (Fig. 1-5). Constricting scar tissue or subcu-

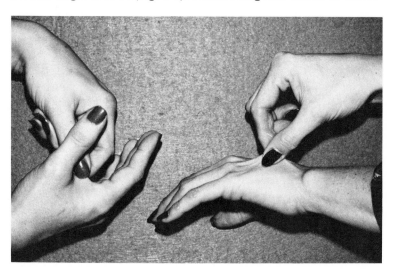

Fig. 1-4. *Tight, tethered volar skin is contrasted with loose, free dorsal skin.*

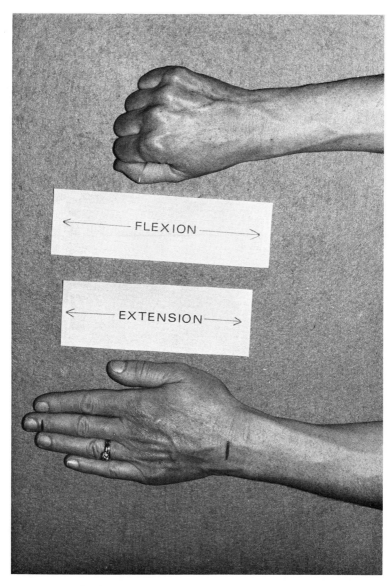

FIG. 1-5. *The length that the dorsal skin must stretch in going from full extension to full flexion is significant.*

taneous edema impairs this flexibility. This can be demonstrated easily by picking up the dorsal skin between the thumb and index finger of the opposite hand and then trying to make a fist; finger flexion is notably restricted (Fig. 1-6).

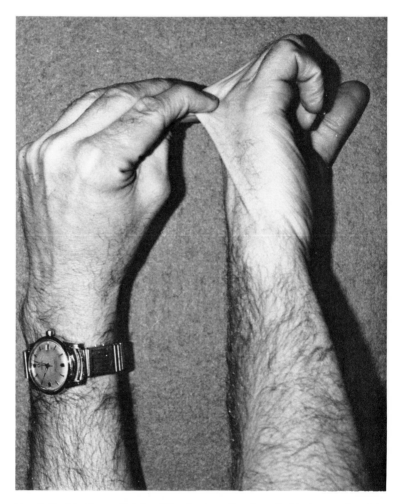

FIG. 1-6. *Making a fist is difficult when the dorsal skin is restricted by another hand, edema, or scar.*

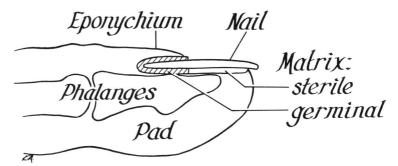

Fig. 1-7. *Cross section of the nail. Nails are extensions of the skin and grow out of pockets that are prone to injury or infection.*

Lying in the loose, subcutaneous, dorsal areolar tissue are the veins and lymphatics—the main drainage system of the hand. Scar tissue, edema, or compression interferes with this drainage. Any venous or lymphatic blockade compounds skin tightness and loss of elasticity. For this reason, the prevention of constriction and edema and the preservation of dorsal veins are vital in primary hand care.

A thin aponeurotic layer lies below the loose dorsal subcutaneous tissues, and under this lie the digital extensor tendons. These tendons are close to the surface. Abrasions, sharp grazing injuries, and burns can easily penetrate the dorsal skin and damage underlying structures. One must assume that any dorsal laceration has damaged the underlying extensor tendons as well until they are visualized intact.

Underlying both the volar and dorsal skin is fat, which is thicker on the volar side. This fat layer provides padding for the hand. It has a tenuous blood supply and it does not regenerate if injured.

The nails are a unique extension of the skin (Fig. 1-7). About three-quarters of the whole nail is visible; the remainder lies in a sulcus that is lined with germinal nail matrix. From this matrix, nail growth occurs constantly. The visible nail is fixed to the finger by the nongerminal (sterile) matrix, which adheres to the distal phalanx. Injuries and infections in this area are common.

The Circulation

The radial and ulnar arteries provide the major blood supply to the hand (Fig. 1-8), in which they form a rich but highly variable anastomotic network. Most hands can survive and function well if one artery or the other is lost. However, in some hands, the loss of

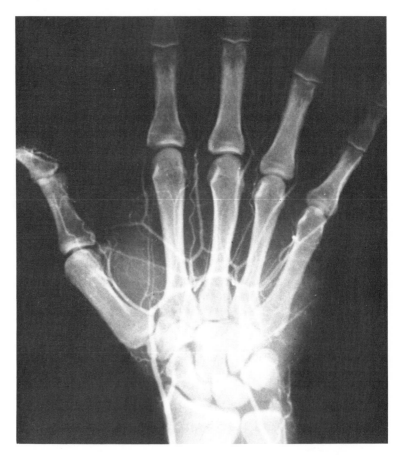

FIG. 1-8. *Radiograph showing the radial and ulnar arteries forming the superficial vascular arch at the "thumb line" level. This arch ramifies into digital arteries.*

one artery will result in necrosis of one or more digits. A simple test to evaluate the relative importance of each vessel in vascular perfusion is the Allen test. To do this test, the examiner compresses the two arteries at the wrist by finger pressure while the patient makes and releases a fist several times to exsanguinate the hand. The patient then holds the fingers in a semiflexed position and the examiner releases the pressure on one artery. The location of the pink flush and the time of its arrival are noted. The test is then repeated with release of the other artery. Careful use of this test will reveal how rapidly and completely each artery perfuses the hand. Filling may be either incomplete (e.g., the ulnar three digits do not fill with radial artery release) or slow, or rapid and equal from each artery.

The radial artery is readily palpated in the distal, radial-volar wrist—the site of the classic "pulse." It usually branches as it enters the hand, giving off a superficial palmar branch while the main branch passes dorsally through the snuff-box (the concavity bordered by the long and short thumb extensors), where it is readily palpable. The superficial palmar branch usually joins the ulnar artery to form the superficial palmar arch. The dorsal branch provides an important branch to the dorsal thumb and goes on to form the deep palmar arch.

The ulnar artery at the wrist is less palpable than the radial artery because it lies beneath the flexor carpi ulnaris tendon on the ulnar-volar aspect of the wrist. It is intimately associated with the ulnar nerve, and injury to one usually means the other has been injured. The ulnar artery passes into the hand to form the important superficial vascular arch. This arch, which gives rise to at least three of five common digital arteries, lies at the mid-palmar level. The level of this vascular arch can be readily ascertained by extending an imaginary line straight across the palm from the volar surface of the fully abducted and extended thumb (Fig. 1-9). The arch crosses the hand at the level of the distal end of the carpal tunnel, just volar to the extensive branching of the median nerve into its terminal sensory branches.

Common digital arteries pursue a course between flexor tendons and superficial to common sensory nerves to the level of the MCP joint flexion crease. At this point the nerves and arteries,

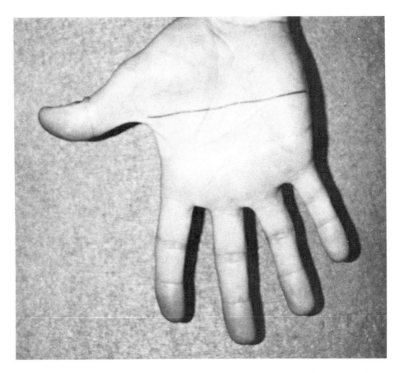

FIG. 1-9. *The "thumb line" or cardinal line is an anatomic landmark to the midpalm level.*

now split into proper nerves and arteries (that is, one to each side of the digit), change position and the nerve becomes more superficial (volar) for the remainder of the digital course. This fact is significant in the diagnosis of digital nerve injury. Blood spurting from a volar finger laceration indicates a lacerated digital artery; since the artery lies deep to the nerve, it almost always indicates a lacerated nerve as well. Digital arteries can often be palpated at the volar base of the finger, about one-third of the way around toward the dorsal surface.

Venous and lymphatic drainage of the hand is extremely important but often neglected. Most of the veins lie dorsally in loose subcutaneous tissue. Constriction from whatever cause (tight sleeves, scars, acute burns, subcutaneous swelling or any other cause) chokes off the low-pressure drainage system and causes a vicious cycle of increased swelling and constriction. Whenever one is treating lacerations, veins should never be heedlessly ligated.

Nerves

Three major mixed motor-sensory nerves need to be considered in the hand: the radial, the ulnar, and the median nerves.

RADIAL NERVE

The radial nerve innervates all of the extrinsic extensor musculotendinous units. (Extrinsic muscles lie in the forearm and their tendons cross into the hand or across the hand into the digits; intrinsic muscles lie entirely within the hand.) The radial nerve innervates none of the intrinsic muscles and plays a relatively minor role in sensibility of the hand.

The radial nerve circles posterior to the midhumerus, enters the forearm above the lateral epicondyle of the humerus and passes through the substance of the supinator muscle. Within the upper one-third of the forearm it gives off all of its muscular branches. The radial-sensory nerve continues beneath the brachioradialis muscle and emerges into subcutaneous tissue on the radial-dorsal forearm about 6 to 8 cm. above the wrist. The nerve branches on the dorsal hand and supplies the dorsal-radial portion of the hand (Fig. 1-10). The nerve is susceptible to compression trauma where it rounds the humerus, and to penetrating or lacerating trauma at any point in its course. Integrity of the motor branch is tested by having the patient extend the wrist, digits II-V at MCP joints, and the thumb at MCP and IP joints (Fig. 1-11).

ULNAR NERVE

The ulnar nerve innervates three extrinsic flexors and 15 of 20 intrinsic muscles, and it provides sensibility to the volar and dorsal aspects of the ulnar side of the hand and the ring finger and to all of the little finger.

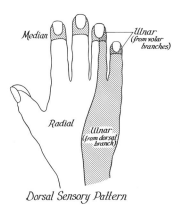

Dorsal Sensory Pattern

FIG. 1-10. *This nerve distribution for dorsal sensory patterns is fairly constant.*

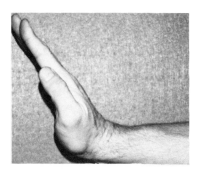

FIG. 1-11. *The motor branch of the radial nerve innervates all extrinsic extensors and can be tested by having the patient extend his hand in this fashion.*

The ulnar nerve enters the forearm through a groove known as the cubital tunnel, which lies posterior to the medial epicondyle. At this point it may be subject to pressure neuropathy. It proceeds along the ulnar side of the forearm deep to the origin of the common extrinsic flexor muscle, and it innervates the flexor carpi ulnaris muscle and the ulnar portion of the common flexor digitorum profundus muscles, mainly those of the ring and little fingers. The nerve then proceeds down the forearm beneath the flexor carpi ulnaris, giving off a dorsal sensory branch about 6 to 8 cm. above the wrist. This dorsal branch supplies the dorsal aspect of the ulnar side of the hand, as well as the proximal dorsal aspect of both sides of the little finger and the ulnar half of the ring finger.

In its course down the forearm, the nerve is accompanied by the ulnar artery and is well-protected by the flexor carpi ulnaris. Nerve and artery enter the hand by way of Guyon's canal, comprising its sole contents. The roof or volar aspect of the canal is formed of thin fascia, fibers of the palmaris brevis muscle and skin. The ulnar border is the pisiform bone and pisohamate ligament. The floor and radial border are one and the same in this triangular-shaped canal, and it is formed of muscle fascia and part of the volar carpal ligament. Just beyond the pisiform bone the nerve gives off volar sensory branches to the little finger and the ulnar portion of the ring finger. These nerves furnish sensibility to the dorsal aspect of the distal phalanges of the entire little finger and the ulnar side of the ring finger. The ulnar digital nerve to the little finger lies in a subcutaneous position on the hypothenar intrinsic muscles. The common digital nerve to the adjacent sides of the little and ring fingers lies between the flexor tendons of these two fingers, with the same nerve-artery relationship discussed previously.

The ulnar intrinsic motor nerve, just after its exit from Guyon's canal, curves around the hook of the hamate bone and travels across the hand between flexor tendons and skeleton, giving off motor branches to all hypothenar muscles, the lumbrical muscles of the ring and little fingers, all volar and dorsal interosseous muscles, and the thumb intrinsic muscles lying to the ulnar side of the flexor pollicis longus tendon. The performance of digital abduction and adduction is a good test for ulnar intrinsic function. A specific test for ulnar motor intrinsic integrity is to observe and palpate the action of the first dorsal interosseous muscle. This muscle is readily palpated along the radial border of the second (index) metacarpal bone. It may be tested by asking the patient to place his hand on a hard surface, lying on its ulnar side. With the examiner holding his index finger on the first dorsal interosseous muscle, the patient is asked to raise his index finger to the ceiling. Contraction of the muscle, or lack of same, is unmistakable (Fig. 1-12).

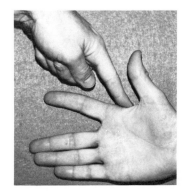

FIG. 1-12. *The ulnar nerve inner-vates 15 of 20 intrinsic muscles. The last one in line is the first dorsal interosseous muscle and its contraction (or lack of same) is unmistakable when the patient is asked to lift the index toward the ceiling.*

Absence of ulnar nerve intrinsic motor function is characterized by a wasted appearance in the interosseous spaces of the
hand and loss of abduction-adduction of digits II through V. In
addition, there is clawing of the ring and little fingers (hyperextension stance of the MCP joints and flexion stance of the IP
joints). Froment's sign is positive (flexion of the thumb at the
interphalangeal joint on forced pinch). This stance is assumed
because, in the absence of the adductor pollicis muscle, the flexor
pollicis longus becomes the primary motor force in pinch.

MEDIAN NERVE

The median nerve enters the forearm adjacent to the brachial
artery beneath the lacertus fibrosis and proceeds down the forearm in the depth of the flexor muscle mass. In its course it passes
between the heads of the pronator teres muscle and innervates
the muscle; this is an area of potential constriction. The flexors
innervated are: the flexor pollicis longus, the four flexor digitorum
sublimi, the radial half of the profundus mass (mainly to the index
finger and long finger), the flexor carpi radialis and the palmaris
longus. At wrist level it innervates the pronator quadratus. Approximately 3 to 4 cm. above the wrist the nerve emerges from
under the muscle mass of the sublimi to lie superficially, covered
only by antebrachial fascia, palmaris longus, and skin. In this area
it is vulnerable to laceration.

At this level of the wrist-palm junction, the median nerve enters
the carpal tunnel in company with the nine digital flexors. The
carpal tunnel extends approximately 4 to 6 cm. from wrist to
midpalm. The thick volar carpal ligament forms the roof of the
tunnel. This ligament stretches between the radial and ulnar sides
of the proximal row of carpal bones, forming a volar concavity.
The ligament is covered by palmar fascia, fat, and thick palmar
skin. This is a common area of nerve compression.

At the distal end of the carpal tunnel, the median motor branch
to the thumb intrinsic muscles branches off and supplies those
intrinsic muscles lying radial to the flexor pollicis longus tendon.
Just distal to the motor branch take-off, the median nerve divides
into sensory branches to the thumb, index finger, long finger, and

radial side of the ring finger, and provides motor branches to the lumbrical muscles of the index and long fingers. This is the level at which the superficial vascular arch crosses the nerve. The sensory nerves then proceed distally in company with their arteries as discussed previously.

The median sensory branches supply the volar portions of the thumb, index finger, long finger and radial side of the ring finger, as well as the dorsal aspects of the distal phalanges of these digits. The median nerve is frequently described as the "eye of the hand" because of the critical need for good sensibility in this portion of the hand (Fig. 1-13).

Testing for sensibility, especially around the nailfold (eponychium) of the index or the long finger, is the best test for median nerve intactness after wrist laceration. The median intrinsic functions are difficult to ascertain accurately, especially in injured patients. The median intrinsic motor nerves include those to the abductor pollicis brevis, the opponens pollicis, and part of the flexor pollicis brevis (thumb intrinsic muscles), as well as branches to the lumbrical muscles of the index and long fingers.

The median-innervated thumb intrinsic muscles are responsible for opposition (or pronation) of the thumb, which enables the thumb to meet the other digits pad-to-pad. When done success-

FIG. 1-13. *The nerve distribution for volar sensory patterns illustrates why the median nerve is known as the "eye of the hand."*

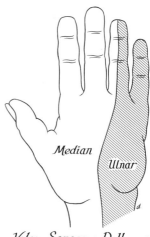

Median

Ulnar

Volar Sensory Patterns

fully, the nails of thumb and opposing digit are 180 degrees apart (Fig. 1-14). Interpreting this test in acutely injured patients is difficult, because it demands good patient cooperation. Also, the ulnar nerve may innervate some muscles normally innervated by the median nerve. Beware of relying on this test. To assess whether or not the nerve is intact, it is far better to rely on tests of median nerve sensibility and/or the location and apparent depth of a laceration. One should remember that the nerve lies only a few millimeters from the skin at the volar wrist.

Loss of innervation of the lumbrical muscles of the index and long fingers results in a mild claw deformity (MCP hyperextension, PIP and DIP flexion) which is subtle and usually noted only by experienced examiners.

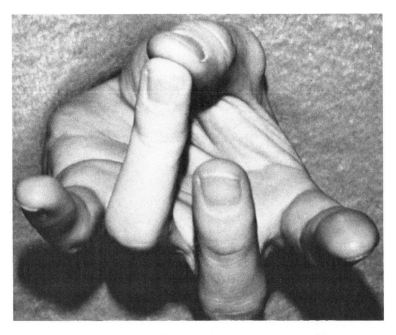

FIG. 1-14. *Median intrinsic function is hard to assess with accuracy, especially in an injured patient. This is how the median-innervated intrinsic muscles turn the thumb over (pronation) to oppose the other digits pulp to pulp.*

Extrinsic Muscles and Tendons

FOREARM MUSCLES

There are few of these muscles, which need to be considered here because of their important function in placing the forearm and hand in positions for optimal function. They pronate and supinate the hand (Fig. 1-15). Five musculotendinous units will be considered—three long muscles and two short muscles with short, broad tendons.

The brachioradialis, innervated by the radial nerve, is readily palpable on the radial aspect of the forearm; it is a powerful elbow flexor and weak forearm supinator. The biceps brachii, innervated by the musculocutaneous nerve, inserts on the proximal radius and acts to flex the elbow, but even more importantly, it supinates the forearm. The supinator is a fleshy muscle, innervated by the radial nerve; it arises from the lateral humerus and the ulna with a broad insertion into the proximal radius across the deep posterior upper forearm. The motor branch of the radial nerve, the posterior interosseous nerve, passes between the two layers of this muscle on its course down the forearm. The pronator teres muscle arises with the common flexor mass and inserts in the midradius. It is a powerful forearm pronator, innervated by the median nerve. The pronator quadratus is a fleshy muscle lying on

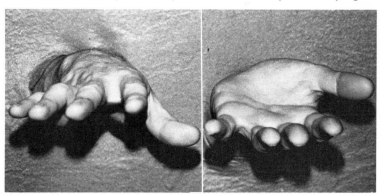

FIG. 1-15. *Pronation (left) and supination (right). These forearm motions are crucial to hand function.*

the volar aspect of the distal forearm between the radius and the ulna. It acts to turn the hand downward into pronation. It too is innervated by the median nerve.

Both the supinator and the pronator quadratus muscles are deeply buried and not accessible to examination by palpation. The biceps and brachioradialis are easily palpated, but the pronator teres is slightly more difficult to palpate.

THE FLEXORS OF THE WRIST AND DIGITS

There are 12 extrinsic flexors. The three that flex the wrist act synergistically with the extrinsic digital extensors. Synergism is an important concept in muscle action. A muscle performs best when it is stretched to a certain degree. In order to stretch digital extensors, the wrist must flex. If the wrist is extended, digital extension cannot be performed with the same strength and completeness that it can with the wrist flexed. Digital flexion acts synergistically with wrist extension. This mechanism can be demonstrated on one's own hand. If one puts the wrist in full flexion and attempts to fully flex the digits, a weak, uncomfortable fist results (Fig. 1-16A). If one extends the wrist, a powerful comfortable fist can be made (Fig. 1-16B). Synergism can be utilized to passively test the intactness of musculotendinous units. If the examiner braces the patient's elbow on a secure platform and moves the wrist from full flexion to full extension, the digits will automatically go from extension to flexion if the musculotendinous units are intact. This is a passive application of synergism, known as the tenodesis effect.

The three wrist flexors, therefore, position the hand so that the digital extensors may work at maximal advantage. The flexor carpi ulnaris, innervated by the ulnar nerve, inserts into the pisiform bone and acts as a flexor and slight ulnar deviator. In its course down the forearm it lies superficial to and protects the ulnar nerve and artery. The other powerful wrist flexor is the flexor carpi radialis, innervated by the median nerve. It inserts more centrally into the second metacarpal base. Its position is just ulnar to the radial artery. Lying just ulnar to the flexor carpi radialis and superficial to the median nerve, which innervates it, is the pal-

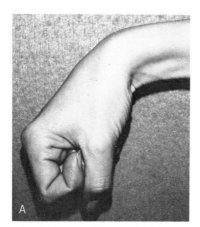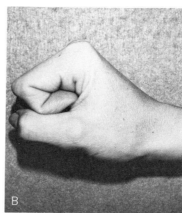

FIG. 1-16. *(A) A tight fist cannot be made with the wrist flexed because the digital flexor muscles are too lax. (B) By contrast, a tight comfortable fist can be made with wrist extended because the digital flexors are stretched just enough.*

maris longus. This is a weak wrist flexor. If it is lacerated, the examiner should suspect median nerve injury, despite clinical evidence to the contrary.

There are nine digital flexors, one for each interphalangeal joint. At wrist level and through the carpal tunnel they are arranged in layers, with the central two digitorum superficialis flexors (to the long finger and the ring finger) on top, the peripheral digitorum superficialis flexors (to the index finger and the little finger) below, and the five profundi flexors and the thumb flexor (to the terminal phalanges) forming the bottom layer. At wrist level the tendons lie in loose areolar tissue with some attached synovium. In the carpal tunnel, they are snugly packed and surrounded by synovium. Upon their exit from the carpal tunnel they lie beneath nerves and vessels in a "free area" (with no fibrous canal surrounding them) for about 2 to 3 cm., and then enter their respective digital thecal sheaths at the level of the distal palmar crease. This is also the level of the metacarpal heads.

Each digital thecal sheath runs from the junction of middle and distal thirds of the palm to the middle of the middle phalanx. It is lined with synovium and has a ligamentous wall of varying thickness. This wall is divided into thin cruciate and thick annular pulleys. At the entrance of each digital thecal sheath, the sublimis lies superficial to the profundus. In the course of the sheath or canal, the sublimis decussates or splits and the profundus moves to the more superficial position, while the two divisions of the sublimis insert into the middle phalanx. The amplitude (glide past a given fixed point) of the tendons in the midportion of this canal may extend to 50 mm.

This canal is the so-called No Man's Land. The term is derived from the admonition of the early days of hand surgery that no man should operate on an acute tendon injury in this area. This concept has changed considerably with the introduction of new techniques, new suture materials, and most importantly, better training in hand surgery. Primary repairs are now performed routinely in this area. Because of the extensive glide of tendons in a tightly enclosed space, infections in this canal may have severe and devastating effects. For the hand surgeon, retrieval of lacerated tendons may present some problems.

Upon its exit from the canal the profundus continues to its insertion at the volar base of the distal phalanx. Both the sublimis and the profundus tendons derive their blood supply from mesenteric-like structures called vinculae. In the event of a laceration, these structures may act as tethers and prevent excessive tendon retraction.

The flexor pollicis longus has a course similar to that of the profundus, but somewhat simpler anatomically because there is no sublimis tendon. The flexor pollicis longus takes a course deep beneath the thenar muscles, which makes recovery after laceration especially difficult.

Testing of the terminal phalangeal flexors (that is, profundi and the flexor pollicis longus) is done simply by asking the patient to flex the terminal phalanges actively (Fig. 1-17). The sublimi are tested by holding all but the finger to be tested in full extension and asking the patient to flex the free finger (Fig. 1-18). This passive extension effectively holds the profundi in full extension and therefore out of action. This is a good test for the long, ring, and little fingers but may not be as accurate with the index finger

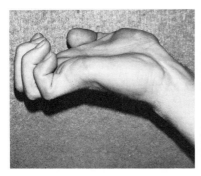 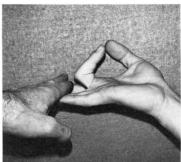

FIG. 1-17. *To test the terminal phalangeal flexors—four profundi and the flexor pollicis longus—ask the patient to actively flex the distal phalanges.*

FIG. 1-18. *The test for sublimis function requires putting the profundi on so much stretch they cannot function.*

because the profundus to the index finger has a certain degree of independence. All of the digital flexors are innervated by the median nerve, except for the ulnar portion of the common profundus muscle belly, which mainly serves the ring and little fingers and is innervated by the ulnar nerve.

EXTRINSIC EXTENSOR TENDONS

There are 12 tendons on the dorsal forearm, wrist, and hand, all of which are innervated by the radial nerve. They act synergistically with the flexor tendons.

Four of these twelve tendons act at the wrist level. Starting at the radial side, the abductor pollicis longus is the first. This tendon stabilizes the base of the first (thumb) metacarpal and deviates the wrist in a radial direction. Although technically not a wrist extensor, this tendon is most conveniently grouped with the extensors. It arises in the midforearm along with its companion, the extensor pollicis brevis. The two move diagonally from ulnar-proximal to radial-distal positions and pass through the first dorsal synovial compartment. (Painful stricture or triggering here is known as DeQuervain's stenosing tenosynovitis.)

The next two tendons are the extensors carpi radialis longus and brevis. They insert into the dorsal bases of the second and third metacarpals respectively. The longus acts as a radial deviator-extensor, while the more centrally inserted brevis acts as a wrist extensor. As they emerge from the second dorsal compartment, they lie deep to the extensor pollicis longus, where that tendon emerges from the third dorsal compartment to move obliquely in a radial direction toward the thumb. The third dorsal compartment is anchored radially on a protuberance of the radius known as Lister's tubercle.

The last of the wrist-level tendons is the extensor carpi ulnaris. It inserts into the base of the fifth metacarpal after emerging from the sixth dorsal compartment, and it acts as an ulnar deviator as well as an extensor.

The three wrist extensors arise on the humerus just proximal to the lateral epicondyle (extensor carpi radialis longus) or from its distal side (extensor carpi radialis brevis and ulnaris).

The thumb is unique in having two digital extensors, one of which acts primarily at the interphalangeal joint. The two tendons, the extensor pollicis longus and the extensor pollicis brevis, cross the radial dorsal aspect of the hand to converge on the metacarpophalangeal joint of the thumb. If the thumb is extended, these two tendons stand out and form a depression between them that is called the anatomic snuff-box (Fig. 1-19). Although brevis and longus join at the MCP joint of the thumb to form a common extensor mechanism, the primary action of the brevis is exerted at the MCP joint, and that of the longus, at the IP joint. The intrinsic muscles also contribute to the extensor mechanism (see p. 26).

Except for the proprius tendon to the little finger, the remaining six digital extensors enter the hand through the fourth dorsal compartment and act primarily at the metacarpophalangeal joints of their respective fingers. Beyond this level they contribute the central slip to the common extensor mechanism or dorsal finger mechanism. They can act as effective interphalangeal extensors only if the metacarpophalangeal joint is held flexed.

Each of the second through fifth digits has a common digital

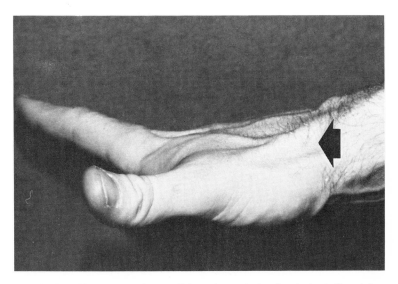

Fig. 1-19. *The anatomic snuff-box (arrow) is the indentation lying proximally in line with the thumb ray at the wrist level. The margins are the extensor pollicis brevis below and extensor pollicis longus above.*

extensor. The second and fifth digits also have an independent extensor called the extensor proprius (indicis for the index finger and minimis for the little finger). The proprius tendons always lie ulnar to the extensor digitorum communis tendons. Occasionally, a long finger may have a proprius tendon as well.

At the wrist level the extensor tendons lie in definite tendon sheaths or compartments with a synovial lining. The amplitude of the tendons is relatively great at this level, and recovery of lacerated tendons is best left to a hand surgeon. Beyond the wrist level there is no tendon sheath; the tendons lie in loose, subcutaneous areolar tissue beneath very thin fascia. The tendons to the second through fifth digits have interconnecting bands called juncturae tendinum. These interconnecting bands so bind the common digital extensors that weak extension of a digit may continue even if the main tendon slip has been divided. Moderate tendon amplitude occurs on the dorsal hand and some retraction may occur with laceration.

The Extensor Mechanism

This unique anatomic entity, also called the dorsal finger mechanism, is a subject of great interest and complexity. Beyond the level of the MCP joint, a combined intrinsic-extrinsic unit extends the interphalangeal joints. The four lumbrical and seven interossei muscles (also known as the central intrinsic muscles), contribute tendons called lateral bands. These lateral bands lie volar to the motion axis of the MCP joints and dorsal to the motion axis of the IP joints; therefore, they act as MCP flexors and IP extensors (Fig. 1-20). The extrinsic extensor tendon continues down the center of the proximal phalanx and inserts primarily in the proximal end of the middle phalanx as the triangular ligament. At this level the lateral bands coalesce and continue to the distal phalangeal insertion. Intrinsic and extrinsic contributions to this common mechanism are held together with ligamentous fibers and form a common unit. The excursion is small, the tendon thin, and laceration may cause a critical change in the balance of the finger.

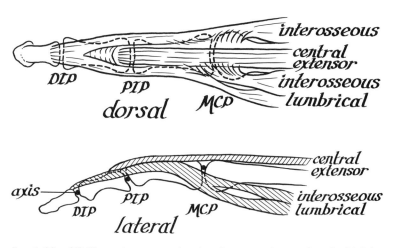

FIG. 1-20. (A) The extensor mechanism is an amalgam of central intrinsic muscles and extrinsic extensors. This view is the dorsal aspect. (B) The extensor mechanism viewed from the radial lateral aspect.

The Intrinsic Muscles

These 20 little muscles, lying entirely within the hand, provide the balancing force between the extrinsic extensors and extrinsic flexors. For convenience, they may be divided into central intrinsic muscles (the interossei and lumbricals), and peripheral intrinsic muscles (thenar and hypothenar muscles). The central muscles form a critical part of the extensor mechanism, as discussed previously. In addition, they adduct and abduct the second through fifth digits. The third digit (long finger) is the central reference for abduction-adduction. Except for the lumbricals of the index and long fingers, all of these muscles are innervated by the ulnar nerve (that is, the ulnar two lumbricals and the seven interossei).

Three hypothenar muscles give the little finger a certain degree of independence with its more mobile metacarpal bone. The thenar muscles are far more important because they give the thumb its great mobility. They are divided into the median-nerve innervated muscles lying radial to the flexor pollicis longus, and the ulnar-nerve innervated muscles lying ulnar to the flexor pollicis longus. The median-nerve muscles are the opponens pollicis, the abductor pollicis brevis, and part of the flexor pollicis brevis. They act to rotate the thumb so its pad can oppose the pads of the other digits at 180 degrees. This action is referred to as opposition or pronation. The ulnar-nerve innervated muscles are a portion of the flexor pollicis brevis and the large adductor pollicis. These muscles give the thumb its power of adduction or the sweep across the palm which is so essential in pinch.

Although these muscles do not often come under scrutiny of the primary care physician, it is impossible to understand and evaluate the hand without understanding their location and function.

Spaces of the Hand

Hand spaces are potential areas of sequestration of purulent material. Two palmar spaces, or bursae, can usually be identified. One is the thenar bursa, which lies between the volar surface of the adductor pollicis and the adjacent long flexors and other intrinsics. The other is the midpalmar space, a potential bursa beneath extrinsic flexor tendons of the long, ring, and little fingers and the underlying intrinsic muscles and bones.

On the dorsum of the hand, a thin aponeurotic layer lies superficial or dorsal to the extensor tendon. Penetrating injuries may cause pockets of purulent material to become trapped in this area.

The flexor tendon sheaths to the thumb and little fingers may be more extensive and reach to the wrist level. A communication between the two across the volar layer of the pronator quadratus muscle is known as Parona's space.

Bones and Joints of the Hand

Unlike central skeletal structures which support body weight, the bones of the upper extremity are designed to maximize the mobility of the extremity while providing adequate support for the primary hand functions of mobility and sensibility.

The hand consists of a series of small bones (carpals) that form a mobile but potentially fixable or stable junction between two series of long bones. These carpals pivot from the two long forearm bones, radius and ulna. In turn, the long, slender metacarpals and the proximal and middle phalanges are cantilevered from the carpals. The long hand bones support the distal phalanges, which bear the fingerpads and nails so critical to hand function (Fig. 1-21).

The *radius* articulates with the capitulum of the humerus. This is a key point of rotation of the forearm bones, which allows the forearm to place the hand in either a supine or a prone position. Distally the radius broadens to form a "seat" for the carpal articulation of the scaphoid and lunate bones.

The *ulna* is quite large at its proximal end where its semilunar notch articulates with the deep trochlea of the humerus to form a secure hinge joint. Distally the ulna ends much diminished in size at the ulnar styloid, slightly proximal to the distal radius. The ulna is attached to the radius by a secure band of fibrocartilage that allows supination and pronation, but it has no carpal articulation.

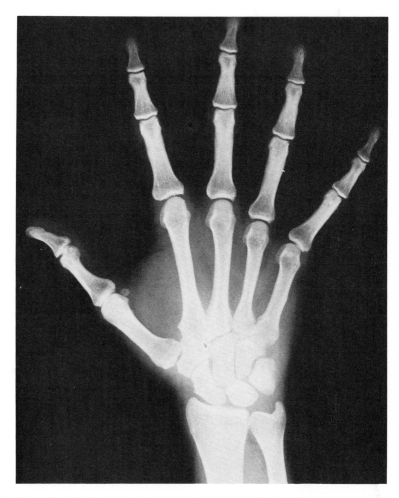

FIG. 1-21. *Radiograph of a normal carpus and hand. The x-ray study is a useful tool in hand injuries. One should have a mental image of the normal.*

The eight *carpal bones* are divided into proximal and distal rows. From radial to ulnar side, the proximal row contains scaphoid (commonly but incorrectly called the carpal navicular), lunate, triquetrum, and pisiform. The scaphoid is a long bone that crosses into the distal row at the level of its waist, where it is vulnerable to injury. It articulates with the radius, lunate, trapezium, and trapezoid bones. Its tubercle is readily palpable in the radial palm.

The lunate is a quarter-moon-shaped bone, as its name implies, with a convex surface against the radius and a concave surface against the capitate. Most wrist flexion-extension movements take place at these articulations. The triquetrum, next in line, has little or no articulation with the radius and serves more to stabilize the ulnar side of the wrist. The pisiform lies in a more volar position and is separate from the other bones. In essence, it is a sesamoid bone serving as an insertion of the flexor carpi ulnaris.

The distal row, from the radial to ulnar side, consists of trapezium, trapezoid, capitate, and hamate. The trapezium has a mobile articulation with the scaphoid. Distally the trapezium forms half of the thumb carpometacarpal or basal joint. This joint is a double saddle, allowing an arc of motion in two directions as well as a certain amount of rotation.

The small trapezoid bone and the large capitate are fixed distally to their respective second and third metacarpals. The hamate forms a somewhat more mobile distal articulation with the fourth and fifth metacarpals.

The carpal bones are strongly supported by ligaments that allow them some mobility but enable the wrist to be firmly fixed.

Projecting from the carpus are the five *metacarpals*. Distally they end in similar hinged joints that allow some abduction-adduction, but mainly permit an arc of flexion and extension. The distal ends of the metacarpals are broader volarly than dorsally. They are attached to the proximal phalanges by firm collateral ligaments that are based dorsally on the metacarpals and in a midposition on the proximal phalanges. Considering the metacarpal shape and the placement of the ligaments, the ligaments are shortest when the fingers are in full extension (Fig. 1-22); if left in this position, the joint will "freeze." Proximally, the metacarpal articulations vary from highly mobile (thumb) to somewhat mobile (little and ring fingers) to quite fixed (index and long fingers).

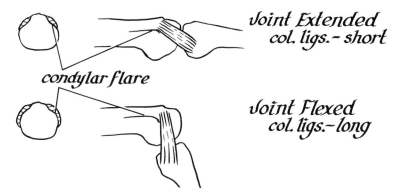

Joint Extended
col. ligs.- short

condylar flare

Joint Flexed
col. ligs.-long

FIG. 1-22. *MCP joints must never be left in an extended position for a long time because the ligaments are the shortest and the joint may freeze.*

The interphalangeal joints are hinged joints, going from 180 degrees extension to between 80 degrees (PIP) and 90 degrees (DIP) of flexion. A firm volar plate prevents much hyperextension and collateral ligaments prevent much lateral motion.

THE INTEGRATED HAND

The hand skeleton forms three arches. In general these permit the hand to form the familiar volar concave position that allows grasp and pinch. The most proximal of these is the fixed transverse arch through the proximal carpal row. Distally a mobile transverse arch runs through the metacarpal heads. Being dynamic, this arch is most subject to reversal by edema, dorsal scars, fracture, and joint fixation.

A single longitudinal arch which is fixed at its proximal end runs from the wrist to the fingertips. It is dynamic at its peak at the third metacarpal head. When the two dynamic arches are in midposition, the hand is in the so-called position of function (Fig. 1-23). Note that the wrist is extended, the MPs and IPs are flexed, and thumb web is open. One should strive to maintain this position whenever the hand must be immobilized. The key joint to obtaining this position is the wrist.

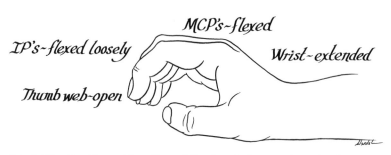

FIG. 1-23.   *Position of function of the hand, the one to strive for.*

The reverse position is called the position of rest-injury (Fig. 1-24). In this position the wrist is flexed, the MPs are extended, the IPs are more tightly flexed (or furled), and the thumb web is closed. Maintaining this position for prolonged periods of time must be avoided.

Integrated hand function depends upon achieving a harmonious relationship among the anatomic parts of the hand. Disease or injury interrupts this relationship. The physician must actively seek to restore the function and not contribute to a budding disharmony by a lack of anatomic knowledge.

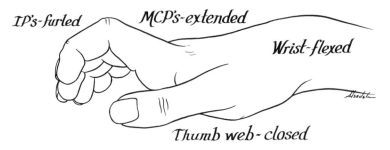

FIG. 1-24.   *The position of rest-injury, to be avoided.*

REFERENCES

1. Lampe, E. W.: Surgical Anatomy of the Hand. CIBA Symposium CIBA Pharmaceutical Co., Summit, N.J., 1969.

2. Kaplan, E. B.: Functional and Surgical Anatomy of the Hand. 2nd ed. Philadelphia, J. B. Lippincott Co., 1953.

2

Diagnosis and Referral of Hand Injuries and Afflictions

M ANY injuries and afflictions of the hand will be encountered in the busy emergency department or office practice. The causes and severity of such problems are as various as the ages, emotional stability, and occupations of the patients. If you get in the habit of following a specific routine when evaluating the hand, the correct diagnosis will be made with greater frequency, and the chances for correct treatment with rapid resolution of the problem will be greater.

The History

GENERAL

Isolated hand injuries rarely present a threat to life and the patient is usually able to give some sort of history. Unless the injury is trivial, it is best to get the patient immediately recumbent on a secure examining table with the hand resting on an attached arm board or other firm support.

It is important to establish hand dominance. When writing down which hand is injured—right or left—add in parentheses whether it is major or minor. It is also important to establish whether there is any prior history of hand disease (most com-

33

monly this would be Dupuytren's fasciitis or contracture, arthritis, or possibly a ganglion or other tumor). Since hand injuries are so common, one should also query the patient about prior injuries and pursue this topic in some detail. Once these three items have been established—hand dominance, preexisting disease, and/or prior injury—one may proceed to elucidate the current problem.

MECHANISM OF INJURY

Establishing the mechanism by which the hand was injured can be helpful in several ways, such as estimating a need for certain diagnostic steps (roentgenograms, blood counts or wound culture). For example, lacerations caused by glass commonly penetrate deeply and should make the examiner automatically suspicious of injury to deep structures. A knife that creases a finger renders less damage than a knife that is grabbed tightly to prevent an assault. A wound sustained in the kitchen obviously has a lesser potential for infection than one sustained in the town dump.

The need for radiographs may be obvious if the hand, or some deep part of it, shows gross deformity. Not so obvious may be the need for roentgenograms if swelling or deformity is minimal; however, if the mechanism of injury suggests a force sufficient to tear ligaments or fracture bones, x-ray examination is mandatory. It is frequently worthwhile to get radiographs of the opposite hand and wrist as well, to put normal variations into proper perspective.

The Examination

PRELIMINARY STEPS

Before any hand can be examined, the patient should be in a stable position, the hand stabilized, and the extremity exposed. Any constrictive or potentially constrictive item of jewelry or clothing should be removed. Be reasonable, of course—it may not always be necessary to bare the patient to shoulder level. Try to avoid any compromise about proper exposure of the extremity and make determined efforts to avoid constriction. Be especially careful of rings, even if they are not on the injured finger. A freely movable ring can become a noose around the finger with just a little swelling.

OBSERVATION

Simple observation is the mandatory first step of the examination. The hand in repose, lying on its dorsal surface, assumes a position of volar concavity with progressively greater flexion from index finger to little finger, as if it were grasping an egg (Fig. 2-1). The thumb lies close to the side of the hand with minimal IP and MCP flexion. Any striking variation from this posture indicates significant abnormality. For example, if the palm is lacerated and one finger sticks straight out, the diagnosis of flexor tendon injury can be made and only dressing and referral are required (Fig. 2-2). In such cases, there is no need to go further with the examination; to do so is unnecessarily meddlesome. At each step ask yourself whether the diagnosis has been made. If it has, then determine whether you are going to treat or refer the patient. If referral is in order, do not further probe, examine, or otherwise tamper with the wound. Manipulation is injury, as is any surgical

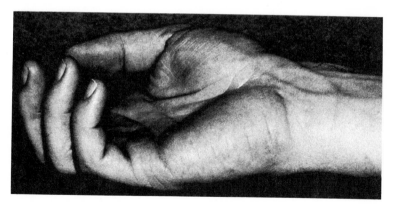

FIG. 2-1. *The uninjured hand in repose. The fingers are loosely flexed as if holding an egg.*

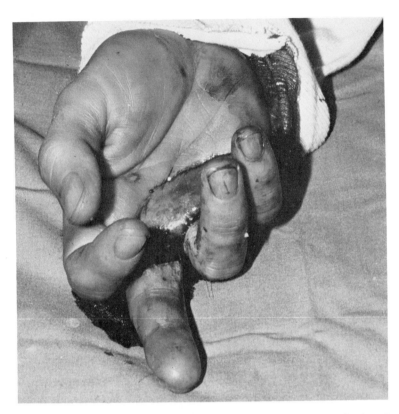

Fig. 2-2.   *The injury is obvious here—nothing but a dressing and referral is required.*

maneuver. As such, it may cause additional swelling, tissue injury, and possible contamination.

The adequacy of the blood supply can be assessed by observing the color of the digits. Gross fractures and dislocations are also apparent on observation.

FUNCTIONAL EXAMINATION

Following observation of the wound and quiescent hand, the next step proceeds to functional examination. As the first maneuver, the examiner has the patient support the elbow on a firm table or support and move the wrist from full flexion to full extension. As can be observed with your own hand, this will move the fingers from extension with wrist flexion to flexion with wrist extension (Fig. 2-3). This is known as the tenodesis effect, and is caused by the passive pull of digital musculotendinous units on one forearm surface as those on the opposite side of the extremity are relaxed. This maneuver demands intact musculotendinous units but no active motion; it is an example of passive synergism (see Chapter 1).

The next part of the functional examination is to evaluate the individual fingers for intactness of tendons. Each flexor tendon is assessed by checking active flexion at each of the IP joints as outlined in the previous chapter. When examining the extensors, remember the mechanism by which the finger extends; avoid

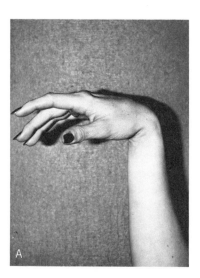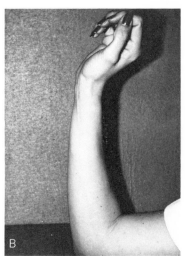

FIG. 2-3. *(A) Wrist flexion causes the digits to extend. This is the tenodesis effect and is an example of synergistic action. (B) The same phenomenon as shown in A, but with wrist extension and digital flexion. Doing these maneuvers passively can give the examiner a lot of information about tendon, bone and joint integrity.*

being fooled by weak but intact extension. Remember that although an extensor tendon may be divided, the finger may be extended by the juncturae tendinum.

If there is any reason to suspect a motor nerve lesion, perform the appropriate test for that nerve. In brief, this entails wrist extension and digit MCP extension for radial nerve function; finger abduction-adduction for ulnar nerve intrinsic muscle function; and thumb opposition-pronation for median nerve intrinsic muscle function (see Chapter 1 for more detail). During these maneuvers, observe the active motion of the joints of any injured part; any abnormality should prompt you to request roentgenograms.

These first two steps involve little or no physical contact with the patient. Obviously, bleeding wounds require dressing, but the greater the exposure of the hand, the better the chance of making a correct diagnosis.

SENSIBILITY TESTING

The third step is to estimate sensibility in areas of possible nerve injury. This is frequently difficult even for experienced examiners. The location of the laceration may be *the* most useful clue to nerve injury. Lack of ability to sweat on a digit distal to nerve injury is proof of a nerve division. It is also a subtle difference that is hard to detect, especially in an acute injury.

In actively examining for loss of sensibility, minimize the maneuvers and perform them when the patient's attention is not diverted otherwise. Use a no. 25 needle to lightly jab suspected areas of decreased sensibility and compare with normal areas. If you suspect nerve injury but cannot be certain, leave the patient alone for a few minutes and then repeat the examination. With suspected loss of the median nerve, the critical area to examine is the nailfold (eponychium) of the index or long finger. With the ulnar nerve, the pad of the little finger is most critical. The area of isolated radial sensory nerve distribution is the dorsal thumb-index web. The first examination and your first impression will be most reliable. Repeated jabbing does little except traumatize the digits being examined.

Laceration of major mixed nerves (that is, the median and the ulnar) demands immediate consultation. Immediate consultation is necessary if the following are lacerated: both nerves in one digit; a thumb nerve; or a border nerve (the radial nerve to the index finger or the ulnar nerve to the little finger). The urgency of consultation is less with other nerve injuries. Some surgeons like to repair nerves at once; others prefer to wait a few days or longer. It is best to establish an understanding with your consultant.

DIRECT EXAMINATION

The fourth step in the examination sequence is direct inspection. Before embarking on this, the arm tourniquet should be in place (see Chapter 3). The hand is prepared for surgery and the area is anesthetized (see Chapter 5). A tray of instruments should be set up (see Chapter 3). Last but not least, you should have a clear idea of the purpose of this inspection. The crucial question is: Is this examination a useful maneuver in terms of diagnosis and treatment, or is it just "poking"? Remember, the more probing or poking that occurs, the greater the chance of causing tissue injury and infection.

Once these preliminary preparations have been concluded, you have to decide whether or not extension of the wound is necessary. It is better to extend a wound surgically than to tear or pull at an edge to visualize the structures. The extension should be done carefully, following accepted lines of incision (see Chapter 5).

In actually exploring a wound, use small skin hooks and retractors (see Chapter 3) to hold the wound open, while gently spreading the soft tissues with fine scissors. If a sound diagnosis and repair cannot be accomplished in 15 to 20 minutes, it to best to desist, close the wound with a few sutures, and refer the patient for more extensive operative exploration and repair.

Factors Complicating History and Examination

The ease of obtaining a history and examining an injury depends on several factors, only some of which are controllable.

The factors that can be controlled to some extent are the surroundings and equipment. A quiet room isolated from the hub-bub of the emergency department, even if only by curtains, is most helpful. Good light and good instruments can greatly ease the task at hand, as can magnification. A tourniquet is essential. (See Chapter 3 for details on these materials.)

Factors beyond one's control include the age, language, and condition of the patient. If time allows, premedication of infants and small children may be a great aid. If this is not possible, it is often useful to anesthetize the injured area, leave the room while the squalling subsides, and then return for direct examination and treatment.

When one cannot communicate with an adult patient because of a language barrier, alcohol or drug intoxication, over-reaction to injury, or any other reason, always assume the worst possibility for a given injury and err on the side of over-referral. Especially in such situations, it is better to probe less rather than more.

Recording Hand Injuries and Afflictions

A concise record of the history and examination is essential. It need not be long but should include written notes on prior injury or disease, mechanism of injury, tetanus immunization status, allergies (especially to antibiotics), which hand has been injured, and which is major.

A hand outline is a useful means to record the examination. Place your own hand on a piece of paper and trace around it with a fiber pen (Fig. 2-4). Your nondominant hand will provide an outline suitable to picture either hand of the patient when it is appropriately labeled right or left, volar or dorsal, ulnar and radial. The wound may be sketched in and tendon and nerve function indicated diagrammatically (Fig. 2-5).

Follow-Up

Every patient should be given access to follow-up. In different communities the doctor to whom the patient is referred may vary

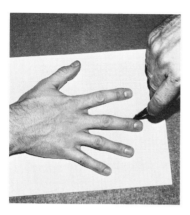

FIG. 2-4. *Making a sketch to record problems discovered during examination of the hand.*

according to specialty, expertise, and competence. The only plea that can be made is that the follow-up physician be a surgeon, hopefully with special expertise in the hand by virtue of training beyond his basic surgical specialty. If this is not possible, then the referred physician should certainly have a special interest and concern for problems of the hand. Random refereal to any orthopedist, plastic surgeon, or general surgeon will certainly result in a

FIG. 2-5. *The entire examination has been diagrammed: there is a laceration at the volar base of the right index finger with loss of sensibility on the radial pad and loss of DIP flexion. This indicates loss of the radial digital nerve and profundus tendon. Such a sketch leaves no room for error or misinterpretation.*

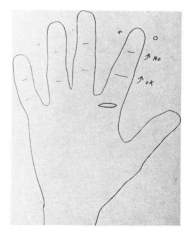

less-than-optimal conclusion. If there is a problem with adequate referral, communication with the American Society for Surgery of the Hand* may be helpful. The Society now has members in most states and has an active educational program.

*Three Parker Place, Suite 233, 2600 South Parker Road, Aurora, Colorado 80014 or check JAMA for listing.

3

Material for Treatment of Acute Hand Injuries

To adequately treat patients with injured hands, one must have specific tools and techniques. Most of the former are easily obtained and relatively inexpensive.

Examining Table and Lights

Patients with hand injuries must be recumbent during examination and treatment (or one may also be treating a patient with a fractured skull when he or she faints). An operating table that can be raised and lowered hydraulically would be ideal, but is not essential. However, the injured hand must be placed on a firm support. This support may be an arm board that attaches to the examining table, or a Mayo stand or some type of small table that can be abutted to the examining table and adjusted to the same height. The hand is placed on this support for diagnosis and treatment. A good light is mandatory: if possible, it should be a "cool" light suspended from wall or ceiling on an adjustable attachment.

Tourniquet

The tourniquet is an accessory that all too often is not used. No hand wound should be examined or treated without benefit of a bloodless field. The pioneer hand surgeon, Sterling Bunnell, observed the following in the first edition of his monumental work:

43

The hand is exceedingly vascular and is filled with tiny structures that will be injured unless our vision is clear and exact. Without a tourniquet our field is ever covered with blood which is opaque . . . Could a jeweler repair a watch immersed in ink?[1]

All hand wounds should be rendered bloodless by means of an arm tourniquet before treatment. This need not be elaborate. For example, one could use a blood pressure cuff placed in the usual position with the tubes pointing cephalad (toward the head) instead of caudad (Fig. 3-1). The cuff is then wrapped with ordinary cast padding such as Webril* or Specialist† (Fig. 3-2), to prevent it from unwrapping when it is inflated. When all else is ready (i.e., anesthesia, skin preparation, and so forth), the patient holds the arm maximally above heart level for 60 seconds. The cuff is then inflated to 250 to 275 mm. Hg. and the tubes (one or both, as the case may be) are clamped near the cuff (Fig. 3-3). Clamping is necessary because the ordinary sphygmomanometer will not maintain this pressure, and the cuff will instead become a venous

*A flat, smooth, cotton flannel material that does not stretch.
†A corrugated cotton flannel material that is stretchable or elastic.

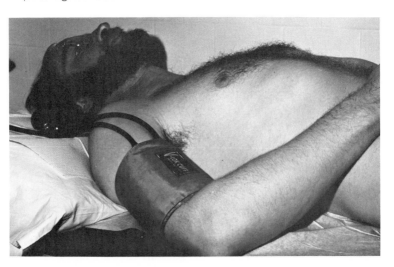

FIG. 3-1. A blood-pressure cuff used as a tourniquet. The entire upper extremity is unencumbered and the tubes on the cuff point cephalad.

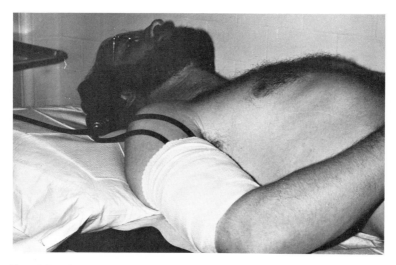

FIG. 3-2.   *Cast padding wrapped around the cuff prevents it from unwrapping in the middle of the procedure.*

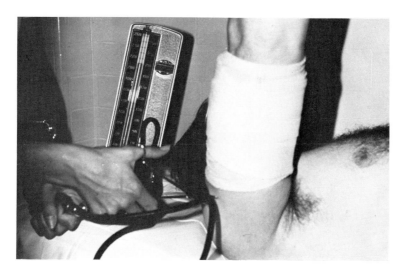

FIG. 3-3.   *The hand is elevated for 60 seconds, and the cuff is inflated to a pressure of 250 mm. Hg. The tubes are clamped to prevent loss of pressure during the procedure.*

tourniquet, making the wound very bloody indeed. Of course, a system designed solely as a tourniquet may be used, but these are fairly expensive and need to have their pressure gauges checked. A cuff from a pneumatic tourniquet set may be purchased separately and attached to the mercury gauge and pump. This eliminates the need for wrapping the cuff, but the tubes must still be clamped.

Patients usually tolerate the tourniquet for 15 minutes; some tolerate it up to 45 minutes with no complaints. In the operating room, with general or regional anesthesia, it is safe for periods up to two hours.

The pneumatic cuff tourniquet is far superior to the rubber-band-around-the-finger method. In this method, a rubber strip is placed at the digit-hand junction and tightly clamped. This causes an undue amount of pressure on end-arteries and veins in an already injured digit. When the rubber strip is removed, deep ridges appear in the skin caused by the constricting force. On occasion, such rubber bands have been inadvertently buried beneath dressings, with predictably disastrous results.

The routine use of rubber band tourniquets is definitely not recommended. If necessary, they should be used only when a patient can no longer tolerate the arm tourniquet but the digital surgery has not been completed—that is, in an already exsanguinated arm. In such a situation, a broad Penrose drain (1.2 cm. to 2 cm.) is applied firmly to the base of the finger. The entire finger is compressed by the surgeon, the drain is clamped, and finally the arm tourniquet is released.

Skin Preparation and Draping of the Hand

Often, as soon as a patient with a wound of the hand arrives in the emergency department, the injured hand is plopped into a basin of an iodine-based or soap-based solution. Virtually without exception, the entire upper extremity is then in a dependent and uncomfortable position and bleeding may continue briskly. This method does little to sterilize the hand and wound, but certainly it frees any bacteria trapped in clots and allows them to enter the wound. It is much better to wrap the wound in sterile dressings and prepare the skin just prior to treatment.

Preparation of the skin may be accomplished with any one of a wide variety of commercially available agents, which include soaps and iodine-based products. A simple, cheap, and proven method is to paint 1% tincture of iodine on the hand and arm up to but not within the limits of the wound. This may be applied with an ordinary paint brush. Alcohol is used to wash the iodine from the skin (Fig. 3-4). Dirty wounds may be flushed with sterile water or

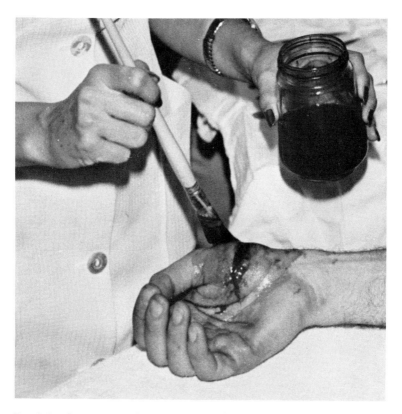

FIG. 3-4.   *One percent tincture of iodine applied around a wound with a paint brush is a useful means of skin preparation.*

saline (or tap water if necessary). The essential idea to remember in wound preparation is that lengthy, vigorous scrubbing is no substitute for meticulous tissue handling and careful postoperative management to prevent swelling (i.e., venous and lymphatic congestion resulting in lack of tissue oxygenation). Debridement and tissue handling are discussed further in Chapter 6.

If a single finger is injured, do not restrict preparation to that finger and then drape it with an eye sheet, as often happens. It is far easier to prepare the whole hand and low forearm and then drape with sterile towels. This makes arm elevation for inflation of the tourniquet easier, and facilitates moving the hand or digit to gain the best exposure. Of course, treating physicians should not have ties, shirt cuffs, or other items dangling dangerously close to wounds.

Magnification

The hand is a relatively small structure composed of many smaller structures. The use of magnification, even in the management of "simple" injuries, is helpful. Magnifying loupes come in a wide variety of shapes, sizes, and prices. A relatively simple, inexpensive device that I have found useful in the emergency department is the Opti-Visor, which can be fitted to any size head (Fig. 3-5). The focal length is only about 8 inches, which is uncomfortable for lengthy procedures but sufficient for short procedures. It gives about 2× magnification. You cannot fully appreciate the benefit of magnification until attempting to do a procedure without it after having used it regularly. I strongly recommend that some magnifying device be available and used regularly.

Instruments

Instruments used in emergency departments are all too often cast-offs from the operating room, and seldom neither delicate nor in good condition. Emergency departments should obtain and carefully maintain a basic set of fine, plastic-surgical instruments

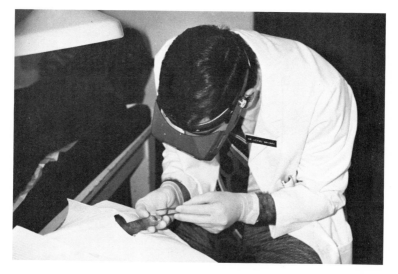

FIG. 3-5.   *Magnification is helpful in doing hand procedures. This is an Opti-Visor loupe.*

because they are essential for proper care of the injured hand. One does not need a large number of instruments, but those obtained should be of high quality and carefully handled. I suggest the acquisition of the following basic instrument set (Fig. 3-6):

1. 1 pair Joseph skin-hooks, 2-mm. gap.
2. 1 pair Ragnell retractors.
3. 1 smooth-jaw Webster needle holder, 10 to 15 cm. long.
4. 1 pair curved, pointed iris scissors, 10 to 15 cm. long.
5. 1 pair straight blunt iris scissors (for sutures) 10 to 15 cm. long.
6. 1 pair single-tooth Adson forceps.
7. 1 small ronguer.

This basic set is supplemented with straight and curved fine mosquito clamps and a knife handle that holds either a No. 15 or No. 11 blade. Other useful instruments that might be added include Joseph skin-hooks with a 4-mm. gap between prongs; small fixation forceps; smooth Adson forceps for applying porous

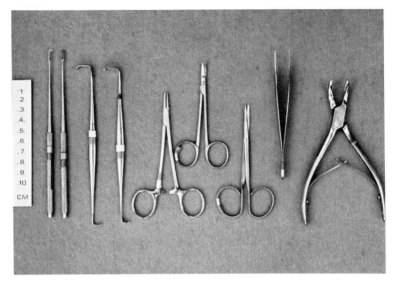

FIG. 3-6.   *These instruments are essential for fine plastic surgery. See text for full listing.*

adhesive paper strips (such as Steri-Strips) or grasping sutures for removal; and other scissors, needle holders, and forceps. The number of instruments is limited only by their cost and the funds available to the department. Many manufacturers of surgical instruments provide catalogs of their wares, whose quality is uniformly good. The names and addresses of specific companies appear in the advertisement pages of such periodicals as *Plastic and Reconstructive Surgery* or *The Journal of Hand Surgery*. These instruments can also be used for plastic repair of facial lacerations and other fine work. If used only for fine work and handled carefully, they will last a long time.

Sutures

The last essential item in the set-up is suture material. In general, suture sizes of 4-0, 5-0, and 6-0 are useful in the emergency room; anything larger than 4-0 material has no place in the hand. A slippery, monofilament, synthetic (nylon) material, such as Dermalon or Ethilon, works best. Braided, nonslippery suture material is not as satisfactory. Blue, green or black sutures are easier to see and handle and therefore recommended, except for tendon suturing. With tendon repair, clear suture material has the advantage of not showing through the skin. (Please refer to Chapter 10.) Absorbable sutures, such as plain catgut or Dexon, are recommended for use in babies and little children because non-absorbable sutures may be more difficult to remove than to insert.

The size and type of needles are as important as the size and type of sutures. Examples of small, curved cutting needles, the proper size for plastic or reconstructive surgery, are P-3 or P-1 (Ethicon) and PRE-2 (Davis & Geck); these are available with suture sizes 4-0, 5-0, and 6-0. The usual 4-0 sutures have FS-2, PS-2, or PRE-4 needles, which are too large for satisfactory fine suturing (Fig. 3-7). Catgut and Dexon are also available with the finer needles.

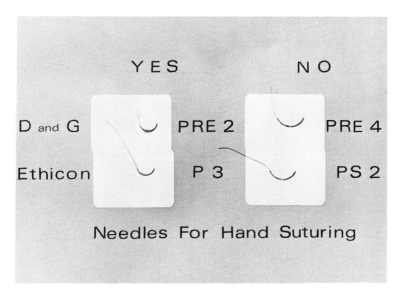

Fig. 3-7. *A comparison of needles showing the sizes required for fine work on the hand.*

The use of the proper equipment and materials greatly enhances the care of the patient with an injured hand. Probably the single most important item is one of the simplest—the use of the tourniquet. Failure to use adequate equipment will lead to treatment that is less than optimal.

REFERENCES

1. Bunnell, S.: Surgery of the Hand. p. 90. Philadelphia, J. B. Lippincott Co., 1944. (Quoted with permission)

4

Dressing the Injured Hand

THE basic purpose of any dressing is to protect an injured part or area against normal wear and tear. Protection implies both cover and enforced immobility. The hand is highly mobile and ordinarily in a dependent position much of the time. Usually the patient wants to use the hand and finds it inconvenient not to do so, especially if he or she is otherwise uninjured and mobile. Any successful dressing must enforce immobility and elevation and provide cover—ultimately, it can be successful only if patient cooperation can be ensured. The patient must understand that it is to his or her advantage to suffer the temporary inconvenience of not using an injured hand.

Fluid Accumulation in the Hand

NORMAL HAND

In normal use the hands are constantly in motion. Thus, although they may be kept below the level of the heart for short periods of time and fairly tight jewelry or clothing may be worn, no special problems with swelling arise. The motion of the hands engages intrinsic and extrinsic muscle units, which forces venous and lymphatic return to prevent swelling. However, mild swelling will occur even in normal hands if they are kept quiet and dependent. For example, mild swelling may occur during sleep, or on long hikes when the hands are held at the sides (possibly aided by compression of axillary veins by pack straps). In an uninjured hand such swelling is overcome by rapidly opening and closing the digits several times. Under normal circumstances, mobility and elevation help to prevent fluid accumulation.

53

INJURED HAND

In an injured hand, fluid exudation inevitably occurs, varying in amount with the severity of the injury. In this situation, activity increases the amount of fluid entering the extracellular space rather than decreasing it, as would occur in a normal hand. Therefore, one of the two natural "antiswelling" mechanisms—mobility—is no longer helpful but harmful. Indeed, it becomes necessary to immobilize the injured hand to prevent further fluid exudation. Thus, the other natural mechanism—elevation—must be used assiduously. In concert with elevation, the absolute avoidance of any constriction of the upper extremity must be carefully observed.

The length of immobilization and the exact position of immobilization depend on the character of the hand and the type of injury. In general, one should put on a larger, more immobilizing dressing than might first seem indicated, but leave it on for a shorter time than might seem warranted. In all cases, the position of immobilization should approach the position of function as closely as possible while keeping the injured tissues quiet.

Immobilization, of course, is a double-edged sword. Besides decreasing fluid exudation, immobilization allows tissues with lacerations, fractures, and other injuries the opportunity to heal in the proper position. However, immobilization should not be prolonged to the point where mobile structures are permanently frozen and rendered useless.

Soft Dressings

WOUND DRESSING

Not only does a nonadherent or minimally adherent dressing next to the wound facilitate wound care, but patients appreciate its ease of removal. This dressing should also allow fluid passage. Xeroform gauze is one such dressing, but others may serve just as well. It is best used as a single layer. Next to the single layer of nonadherent dressing, four to eight thicknesses of soppy wet surgical sponge are used. In emergency departments or physician's office, tap water may be used to wet the sponge; sterile water, saline, or Ringer's lactate are often used and serve well. The wet dressing serves to facilitate movement of blood out of the wound and into the dressings by hydrostatic action. Even under a cast the dressings will become totally dry in three to four days.

Before applying a circumferential bandage, a foam sponge layer about 3/16 inch (5 mm.) thick is placed over the other dressings as a protective layer that allows compression without constriction. Reston is an excellent compressible spongy material with one nonadherent surface and one adherent surface backed with removable paper.

The digits or hand is next wrapped with a "springy" type of coarse-meshed gauze such as Kling or Kerlix. This should never be put on with constricting force. Some physicians like to use tubular elastic gauze that is applied with a wire cage (Tube Gauze), which is fine if one is careful to avoid creating a tourniquet effect with the application of successive layers. The inclusion of a finger adjacent to the injured one in the dressing facilitates application of the dressing and immobilization.

ZINC OXIDE

A variety of opinions exist about how to treat a wound that should remain open—such as an opening to an abscess cavity. One method is to soak the wound several times a day, but the patient may experience difficulty with the dressing. Zinc oxide ointment, which is readily available, provides an excellent answer to this problem. Zinc oxide ointment is hygroscopic: it draws fluids from wounds and skin and by so doing it acts to keep wounds open and to loosen debris. It should be applied generously (Fig. 4-1); wounds may be dressed occlusively and inspected only every second or third day. Minor skin maceration may occur but this is not a short-term problem, and zinc oxide ointment is used only for short terms (eight to ten days).

CORE DRESSINGS

One of these dressings covers the wound and constitutes the *core* dressing. In the care of a small peripheral wound, a core

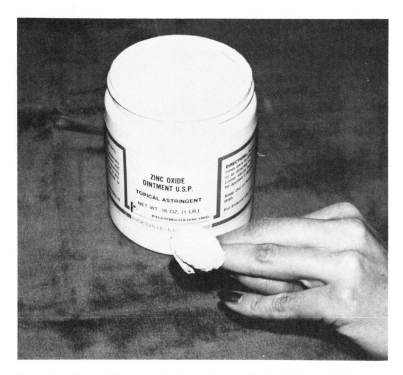

Fig. 4-1. *Zinc oxide comes in large jars and should be applied generously.*

dressing may suffice, but far more often a *shell* dressing of plaster in some form is indicated.

Use of Plaster

GENERAL PRINCIPLES

A well-known aphorism in hand surgery, attributed to the late L. D. Howard, is "Everything heals faster under plaster." With plaster, one can make an infinite variety of casts and splints with the common advantage of being adapted to the patient rather than having the patient adapt to the cast.

The use of circular plaster to dress acute injuries has an unde-
served bad reputation for being constrictive. *Any* circumferential
dressing may be constrictive and dangerous if incorrectly applied,
or if the patient fails to heed carefully given instructions. However,
the exigencies of the times, as well as many local situations,
dictate against the use of circular plaster for casts or splints. This
is unfortunate because nothing protects quite as well as a circular
plaster dressing. Because I firmly believe that it is important to
know how to use both plaster casts and splints for the hand,
directions for making these follow.

SHELL DRESSINGS

One must think of circular plaster as a plaster shell or plaster
dressing rather than as a cast. Cast padding is wrapped on top of
the core dressing. Specialist cast padding is my first choice because of its corrugated construction and "springiness." Webril,
which is flat and unyielding, is my second choice. Two to four
layers of padding are used; these should cover about one-half to
two-thirds of the length of the forearm for most hand injuries. As
discussed in the section on synergism in Chapter 1, wrist motion
automatically causes finger motion, and therefore, true digital
immobilization is possible only with wrist immobilization. The only
exceptions to this rule occur with certain injuries to the PIP and
DIP joints. After application of the cast padding, a three- or four-
inch wide plaster splint of six to eight thicknesses and appropriate
length is dipped in warm water and placed along the volar (or, if
indicated, dorsal) aspect of the full length of the proposed cast. A
central strip running the full length of the cast is then elevated as
a *keel*, which gives greater strength per unit weight to the structure than flat plaster.

The cast is then completed by the application of circular plaster. Usually one or two rolls of three-inch plaster suffice. As the
plaster sets, one should do the final positioning of the wrist and
digits to assure the desired position. The use of warm water and
one of the fast-set plasters greatly speeds up the time in which the
plaster hardens. During the application of the cast the patient's
elbow should be firmly fixed on a solid table or stand to prevent

working on an unstable, moving object. With any cast, complaints about throbbing pain should dictate splitting or removal of the cast. Careful monitoring of pain is far more important than observation of the digits.

THE BOXING-GLOVE CAST

A type of cast that is useful for any injury in which the entire hand needs to be dressed occlusively is the boxing-glove cast. Burns, severe crushing injuries, or even less severe injuries in unreliable patients or children are types of injuries and patients on whom it may be used.

The same concept of core and shell dressings applies. The wound is dressed appropriately and then a sopping wet gauze bandage (Kerlix) is placed in the palm. The fingers and thumb are molded around it in the position of function. A piece of foam sponge (Reston), $\frac{3}{16}$ inch (5 mm.) thick, is applied over gauze on the entire dorsal hand and up the forearm. This is wrapped with cast padding. Plaster is wrapped around the entire hand up to the upper one-third of the forearm. With babies or small children, it is best to make this a long-arm cast because they are so adept at getting out of short-arm casts. This cast provides excellent, comfortable protection. Again, throbbing pain merits immediate attention.

CUSTOM-MADE SPLINTS

Splints are almost as useful as a plaster shell. To fashion one type of splint, make a keeled volar splint as described previously, but use bias-cut stockinette instead of circular plaster to wrap the splint to the extremity. In such a situation, make the splint a bit thicker, using 14 to 16 layers of plaster instead of 6 to 8.

Figure 4-2 demonstrates the construction of a common splint. Cut a sufficient length of foam sponge (Reston) that is $\frac{3}{16}$ inch thick (5 mm.). Cut out to make the desired shape, being certain that the nonadherent side is next to the patient's skin when cutting the pattern. Remove the protective backing of the Reston from the adherent side, and apply a layer of smooth cast padding

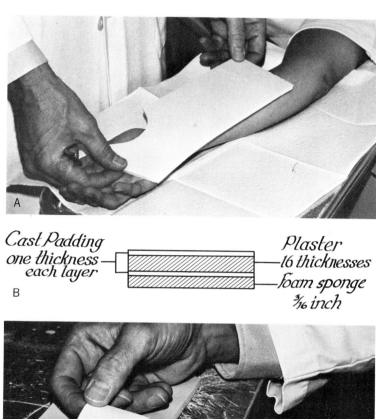

Cast Padding
one thickness ——
each layer
B

Plaster
—16 thicknesses
—foam sponge
3/16 inch

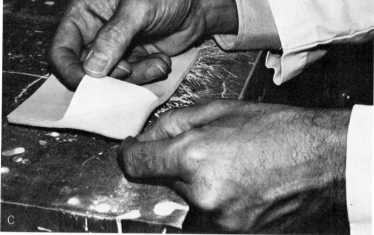

FIG. 4-2.   (A) Cut the foam sponge (Reston) to an appropriate pattern.
(B) A well-tested formula for splint construction. (C) Peel back the
protective paper of the Reston foam sponge to expose the sticky surface.

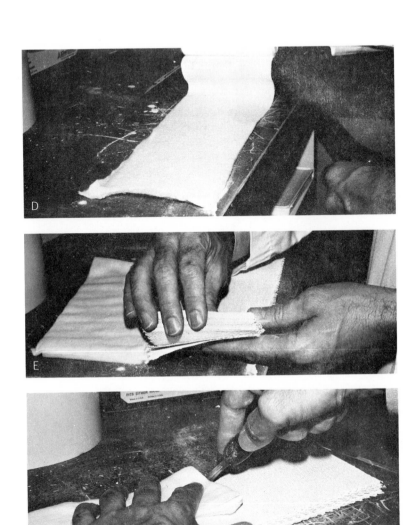

FIG. 4-2. (Cont'd) (D) Lay smooth cast padding (Webril) on the sticky surface of the Reston in a double layer. The plaster will be sandwiched between layers. (E) Count out 16 thicknesses of plaster. (F) Trim the plaster to the Reston pattern. A large knife and cutting board are useful but not essential for this purpose.

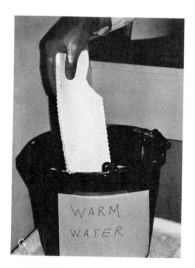

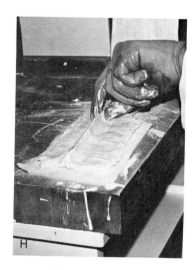

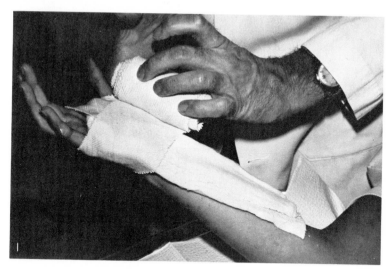

FIG. 4-2. (Cont'd) (G) *Warm water makes the plaster set quickly.* (H) *Make a "keel" in the plaster to give the cast more strength per unit weight.* (I) *Apply the splint and hold it in place with bias-cut stockinette or an elastic bandage. An infinite variety of shapes is possible, all tailored to the patient's needs.*

(Webril) rather than corrugated padding (such as Specialist) to the sticky surface. Then cut 16 thicknesses of plaster to the Reston pattern. This is done most efficiently with a large surgical knife on a cutting board. Dip the plaster in warm water, make a keel, and cover the plaster with another single layer of cast padding. Apply the splint to the digit-hand-forearm. Final positioning of the hand can be done as the plaster dries, while the extremity is stabilized by supporting the elbow on a table or stand. To hold the splint in place, wrap with bias-cut stockinette or elastic bandage such as Ace. The danger of constriction is less with stockinette, but elastic bandage may be used if not wrapped too tightly. This type of splint may be used for an acute injury and also for problems such as a sprain or a carpal tunnel syndrome that is not being treated surgically. Because this splint may be cut to any pattern, it is truly custom-made and fits perfectly. Another advantage is that it may be removed and reapplied by the patient.

Nonplaster Splints

READY-MADE FOREARM SPLINTS

Ready-made splints similar to the plaster ones just described are available. However, they are invariably too big or too small and often uncomfortable. Because the plaster splint is easily made and totally suited to an individual patient's needs, it is far preferable. Ready-made splints may be applicable in mass-casualty situations; otherwise, they are decidedly inferior for upper extremity immobilization.

DIGITAL SPLINTS

The use of aluminum or wooden splints that cross PIP, DIP, and MCP joints, and end at the midpalmar level is common. When one considers the mechanics of the hand (see Chapter 1, especially synergism), the use of such splints does not make much sense (Fig. 4-3). Isolated immobilization of an IP joint is reasonable and possible, but immobilization of a single MCP joint is not practical without immobilizing the wrist. If an MCP joint needs to

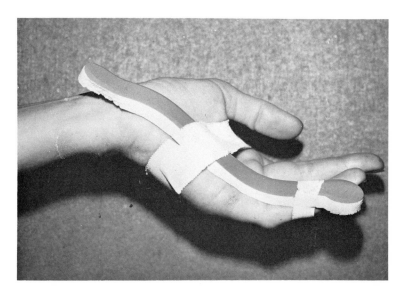

FIG. 4-3.   *The design of this kind of splint does not take into account the mechanics of hand function, and therefore it is not a good splint.*

be immobilized, it is far better to make a digit-hand-forearm splint.

A wide variety of splints are manufactured just for use on digits. These splints fall into two general categories: (1) single-surface, padded splints, sometimes with extensions that wrap around the digit to hold them in place; (2) four-prong, padded or unpadded, malleable splints. These are really guards rather than immobilizing splints. The first type can be easily made by cutting a tongue blade to the appropriate length and covering it with sponge foam (Reston). It is then taped in place. If one uses the commercially available foam-backed metal splints, they should be flat and straight and a pair of tin snips should be at hand to cut them to the appropriate size. Splints with various curves and angles that are difficult to cut to size are not useful. A splint especially to be discouraged is the Freddy-Frog (Fig. 4-4). It is supposed to hold the digit in an uncomfortable position (PIP flexion and DIP hyperextension) that cannot be maintained and is

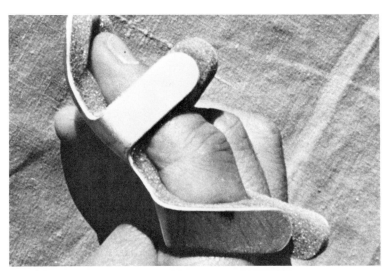

FIG. 4-4. *The design of this splint forces the digit into a position that might cause vascular compromise. It is not recommended for use.*

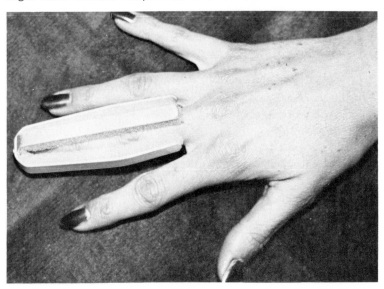

FIG. 4-5. *This four-pronged padded splint is useful for protecting the digit but not for truly immobilizing it.*

unnecessary. The proper splinting for DIP joint injuries is discussed in the section on mallet fingers.

The four-pronged splints are useful for protection of an injured nail, nailbed, and fingerpad (Fig. 4-5). They are especially useful in follow-up care after the acute phase of injury has subsided, because the patient can take them off and replace them for personal hygiene activities such as hand washing and showering.

Elevation of the Injured Hand

Elevation may be achieved in whatever way is easiest and best for the patient. If he or she will walk around with the forearm resting on top of the head (and a few will), that is fine. Most

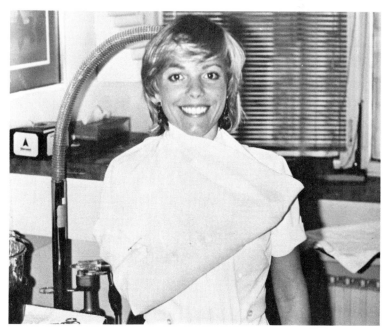

FIG. 4-6. *A sling should hold the hand at heart level or higher. The triangular muslin bandage is excellent for this purpose. Pinning the sling behind the neck is more comfortable than tying it.*

people need some help and for them a properly applied sling is appropriate. The best type of sling is an old-fashioned triangular bandage adjusted to hold the injured hand, resting at heart level or a little higher (Fig. 4-6). The sling will be much more comfortable if it is pinned rather than tied at the back of the neck. At home the patient can support the extremity on a pillow when in bed. Slings that do not permit elevation to heart level are worse than useless and should never be used.

Aftercare

The purpose of any dressing, cast, or splint is to protect and immobilize an injured part so that maximal healing can take place in the shortest time with maximal patient comfort. No immobilizing dressing should be left on so long that parts become stiff beyond redemption. In general, in the hand, this means less immobilization time rather than more. The doctor should keep in close touch with the patient, even if only by phone, to make certain that swelling is minimal and discomfort mild. Throbbing pain under any circumstance indicates a mechanical problem, and inspection of the extremity rather than additional analgesia is mandatory. It means that something—whether cast, splint, dressing, skin, or fascia—is too tight, and mechanical relief must be rendered.

Dressings should be tailored to the individual patient and his or her needs for a given affliction. No dressing, cast, or splint is better than its maker. A high quality in the construction and application of dressings, casts, and splints comes from understanding what is required and then practicing making and using them.

5

Ancillary Measures in Acute Hand Problems

THIS chapter concludes Part I on the Basic Essentials of Hand Care. It is comprised of short discussions of topics that are important to the successful resolution of injuries of the hand: the use of regional and local anesthesia in emergency care of the hand; suitable incisions; the definitive and prophylactic use of antibiotics; tetanus prophylaxis; and the responsibilities of the patient and the physician in the treatment of hand injuries.

Principles of Anesthesia of the Hand

There are two general rules about anesthesia of hand injuries in the emergency department: always use it, but never with epinephrine.

If pain could be quantitated, the pain of placing one or two sutures might approximate that of placing a local or a digital anesthetic. However, when you are placing fine sutures with exactness, you should not have to fight a patient who is jerking his hand because of pain. It is far better to have the area anesthetized. The same thing applies with "trivial" procedures, such as perforation of a nail for a subungual hematoma. Always ask yourself the question: "Would I want an anesthetic if it were my hand or my finger?"

Local anesthetics containing epinephrine are used for two reasons: (1) to reduce bleeding in the wound; (2) to prolong the duration of the anesthesia. By following the principles outlined in

67

Chapter 3, especially the admonition about always using a tourniquet, the wound or incision is rendered bloodless far more effectively than with the use of epinephrine.

Ordinary lidocaine provides about 15 to 45 minutes of effective anesthesia, depending on how (infiltration vs. nerve block), where (digit vs. wrist), and in what strength (1% vs. 2%) it is used. Procedures that require more time than this for their completion are by definition too extensive to be handled in the office or emergency department. In a situation of that magnitude, the patient should be referred to the consultant for treatment in an operating room.

Thus we must conclude that there are no valid reasons for using epinephrine in the lidocaine for anesthesia in primary hand care. However, there is one good reason for not using it: epinephrine causes arterial spasm, and when it is injected next to an end-vessel, it may cause enough spasm to compromise the viability of the digit. Do *NOT* use lidocaine with epinephrine in the hand.

ANESTHETIC AGENTS AND STRENGTHS

Lidocaine is the agent usually available, especially under the trade name, Xylocaine. Other longer-acting agents are used by anesthesiologists, but in general, they have no place in emergency room treatment. Usually lidocaine is used in the 1% strength; for a wrist block, 2% is probably better. Systemic reactions occur only with intravascular injection or with doses over 50 ml. Neither of these situations will prevail in primary care of the hand if a modicum of care is exercised. The minimal amount of the agent to achieve the required end is the correct amount. Avoid injecting so much solution that the tissues become tense and congested from the bulk of fluid.

NEEDLES FOR ANESTHETIC INJECTION

The ideal needle for all wrist, hand and digit blocks is the $\frac{1}{2}$-inch (12.5 mm.) no. 27. A no. 30 needle is a bit too flimsy, but a no. 25 needle serves quite well. No nerve lies more than 6 to 8 mm. below the surface, so a needle longer than ½ inch (12.5 mm.) is not necessary. Needles larger than no. 25 are unnecessary to deliver the required volume, and they may lacerate nerves more easily owing to their large size.

The two basic types of anesthesia are regional block and local infiltration. Local infiltration anesthesia has limited use in the hand. It should be used only where the skin is fairly loose (i.e., the dorsal hand), or in very small palmar lacerations. The solution should be used in small amounts. The needle should be introduced into the subcutaneous tissue through the wound rather than through a series of separate stab wounds.

REGIONAL BLOCKS

The hand is particularly well-suited to regional blocks because the nerves are isolated with good identifying landmarks and lie close to the skin. The syringe is handled and needle introduced as shown in Figure 5-1.

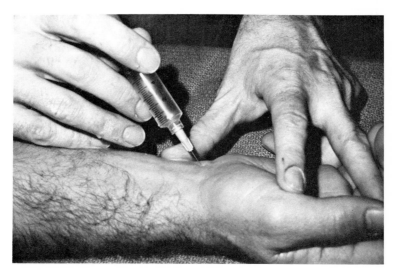

FIG. 5-1. *This shows the correct way to hold a syringe while inserting the needle.*

WRIST BLOCKS

There are four possible wrist blocks; a review of Chapter 1 will be helpful in locating the nerves.

The radial nerve emerges from beneath the brachioradialis tendon about 6 cm. above Lister's tubercle. Infiltration of the subcutaneous tissue over a 2-cm. wide band, about 2 cm. below this point, will block the nerve (Fig. 5-2).

The dorsal sensory branch of the ulnar nerve comes off the main ulnar trunk about 6 to 8 cm. above the ulnar styloid. It may be blocked by 3 to 4 ml. of solution placed subcutaneously over a 3-cm. breadth about 4 cm. above the styloid. This block is infrequently used.

The main ulnar trunk provides volar sensibility to the little finger and ulnar side of the ring finger as well as intrinsic power to 15 of 20 intrinsics; it lies just beneath the easily palpated flexor carpi ulnaris in the distal forearm. An examination of your own extremity will reveal how easily the flexor carpi ulnaris becomes apparent on wrist flexion. Introduce about 2 ml. of solution first from the ulnar side and then 2 ml. from the radial-volar side of the tendon. Take care to be certain that you have not entered the ulnar artery (Fig. 5-3).

Block of the ulnar nerve at the elbow is sometimes advocated. Here the nerve goes through a tight tunnel, the cubital tunnel, beneath the medial epicondyle. Blocks in this area may permanently damage the nerve, either by causing undue pressure or direct laceration. I recommend that this area be avoided for ulnar nerve block.

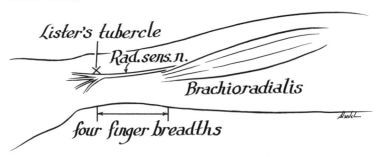

FIG. 5-2.   *Landmarks for a radial sensory nerve block.*

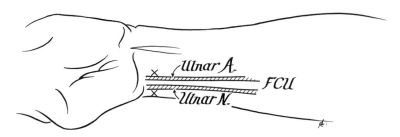

FIG. 5-3. *If you flex your wrist and extend your digits, the flexor carpi ulnaris tendon (FCU) stands out nicely. Avoid injecting into the ulnar artery.*

The median nerve lies deep to the gap between the palmaris longus and flexor carpi radialis tendons (Fig. 5-4). Skin and antebrachial fascia are its only protective covering at this area. It may be readily blocked with about 4 ml. of solution. While instilling the solution, place your opposite thumb just proximal to the needle to force the solution into the carpal canal (Fig. 5-1). This is the same technique used in treating a carpal tunnel syndrome by the injection technique.

DIGITAL BLOCKS

There is no single best way to block digital nerves. The most important thing to know is the anatomic position of the nerves,

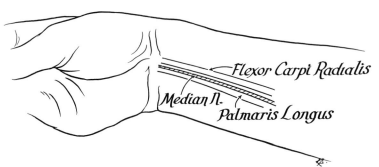

FIG. 5-4. *Landmarks for a median nerve block; the nerve lies close to the skin.*

and base whatever block is selected upon this knowledge (Fig. 5-5, 5-6).

A useful type of block is shown in Figure 5-5B. The needle penetrates the skin only once and is placed first on one side and then the other side of the digit for deposit of about 0.5 to 1.0 ml. of solution on each side. If the proximal two-thirds of the dorsum needs to be blocked, a wheal of anesthetic is raised across the dorsal finger just distal to the MCP joint.

If adjacent digits are to be blocked, the common sensory nerve may be approached in the valley between the flexor tendons to the two digits about 2 cm. proximal to the MCP flexion crease.

The volar digital nerves to the thumb lie much closer to the midvolar surface than do those on the other digits. The MCP flexion crease is the landmark. A rather broad dorsal wheal should be raised on the thumb to ensure a complete block. The dorsal infiltration of any digit should never use more than 2 to 3 ml. of solution.

Sufficient time should be allowed for blocks to "set" before elevating the tourniquet and starting exploration or surgery. For a wrist block, allow 20 minutes; for a digital block, ten minutes.

OTHER ANESTHESIA

Some will advocate more proximal blocks, such as the axillary block, or total blocks, such as intravenous lidocaine. These have

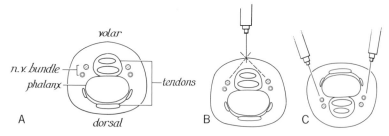

FIG. 5-5. A knowledge of anatomy is crucial to successfully performing regional anesthesia. (A) Cross section at the MCP flexion crease showing access for digital block. (B) A useful volar approach that requires a single penetration of the needle. (C) Many surgeons prefer this approach, but two penetrations with the needle are needed.

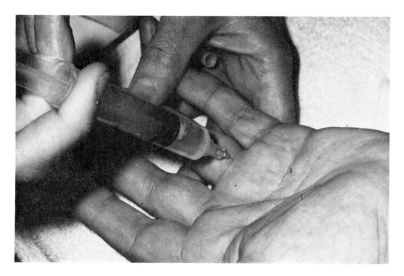

FIG. 5-6. *This shows the technique I use for digital volar blocks.*

no place in the emergency department in the diagnosis and treatment of hand injuries. Likewise, topical anesthesia, such as ethyl chloride spray, has no place in hand treatment.

Incisions

Situations will arise, although infrequently, when it is either desirable or necessary to make an incision on the hand. Types of incisions vary widely from surgeon to surgeon, but certain general principles prevail.

1. Never cross a flexion crease at a right angle on the palmar surface of digit, hand, or wrist. It is acceptable to come up to, but not across, a flexion crease. This rule will be emphasized several times in the treatment of specific injuries.

2. On the dorsum of the hand, the skin is much looser and scar contractures do not pose such a serious problem.

3. When a wound requires extension or when incision is necessary, it is best to trace the incision prior to actually incising. This

may be done with a sterile marking pen or a dye, such as methylene blue, applied with a sharpened applicator stick.

4. When extending a wound, decide where access is needed
and then draw a line proximally or distally from one corner of the
wound as needed. Acceptable lines of incision are shown in Figure
5-7.

5. Always think about what structures lie under any proposed
incision and avoid them assiduously. Always use the tourniquet.

Antibiotics

Discussion of the pros and cons of prophylactic antibiotics is
unlikely to be quelled by dispassionate evidence. There is no
question that antibiotics are unable to overcome the effects of
rough, gross surgery, or post-traumatic and postsurgical swelling.
However, in the untidy injury they may turn the tide against
infection. I recommend that antibiotics be used liberally and early.

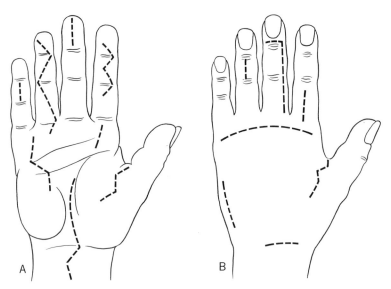

Fig. 5-7.   (A) *Some possible volar incisions. Don't cross flexion creases
at right angles. (B) Useful dorsal incisions.*

The sooner antibiotics are administered after an injury the more good they will do. For practical purposes this means giving the first dose (and hopefully, medication for two or three more doses) in the emergency department.

Some hand infections, mainly streptococcal, are caused by gram-positive organisms susceptible to penicillin, and this is the drug of choice. For apparent staphylococcal infections, initiate treatment with one of the synthetic or semisynthetic penicillins. In case of penicillin allergy, use erythromycin or an oral cephalosporin, but be aware of the kinship between penicillin and cephalosporins in patients who are highly sensitive to penicillin. In major crush injuries that are untidy, use cephalosporins.

A high-loading dose followed by maintenance doses for three or four days is the usual schedule for administering prophylactic antibiotics. See Chapter 9 for further discussion about antibiotics.

Tetanus Immunization and Prophylaxis

Standard practice should be followed here. A tetanus toxoid booster injection should be given if more than five years have passed since the patient received the last booster. Unimmunized persons require passive immunity with injection of human tetanus antitoxin (such as Hyper-Tet); active immunity with tetanus toxoid injection should be started, although it will have no effect on possible tetanus infection of the current wound. The patient must receive instructions on completing the active immunization series. In patients whose last toxoid booster was received more than five years ago, human tetanus antitoxin may be given for tetanus-prone wounds (such as barnyard injuries), as well as injection of tetanus toxoid booster.

Responsibility for Care and Follow-up

PHYSICIAN RESPONSIBILITY

The primary care physician in an emergency department or private office must determine the extent of treatment that he or she can render to patients with injured hands. Whether one should treat the injury definitively, or treat minimally with referral to a hand specialist, or forgo treatment altogether and refer the patient to a specialist for immediate attention depends on several factors. First and foremost is the magnitude of the injury. If the injury is such that definitive treatment in the emergency department or office is feasible, the treatment that you render will depend on the availability of expert help and your own training, experience, and inclination. It would probably be foolhardy for an emergency care physician or family practice physician in a large metropolitan medical center to undertake repair of an extensor tendon when hand surgeons are readily available. By the same token it seems unnecessary to send a patient in a remote area many miles for treatment if the attending physician has the tools and experience to repair the injury. Probably the most important points are that you accurately assess your own abilities, render only treatment that is accepted as standard in your community, and do not undertake procedures with which you are uncomfortable or unfamiliar.

Having rendered competent medical care with a modicum of sympathy, you owe the patient an explanation of what is wrong, what may be expected regarding further treatment and time of recovery, where to secure necessary follow-up treatment, and how to care for the hand in the interim. Your explanation of the disorder should be kept as simple and straightforward as possible. Predictions regarding the time of recovery and possibility of further treatment should be kept as general as possible. Avoid committing a subsequent attending physician or surgeon to a course of action that he or she cannot follow. Referrals for follow-up treatment will vary according to the community; suggestions for follow-up care are discussed at the end of Chapter 2.

Instruct the patient carefully about keeping the injured hand elevated, protected from water, and as inactive as possible (UP, DRY, and QUIET). The patient has to understand that these instructions are important and that it is his or her responsibility to follow them.

Patients are usually given mild analgesics and sometimes antibiotics. The exact function of these medications and the timing of administration should be explained.

Many patients with injured hands are entitled to worker's compensation benefits. Although such laws vary from state to state, it is your responsibility to make sure that the proper forms are completed and submitted promptly. This will ensure both payment of your fee and institution of compensation benefits to the patient.

PATIENT RESPONSIBILITY

Following any injury, patients display an almost universal desire to turn the clock back to one second before the accident and to rearrange subsequent events. Patients may articulate this impulse in just that way, or they may express it in other ways, such as showing anger at their job, their boss, or you, the doctor. The patient may try to bargain with you about the necessary treatment, the dressing, or even more trivial matters. Generally patients try to minimize the seriousness of the injury; the rationale is that if the treatment is minimal, the injury must be minimal too. I have never been satisfied with the subsequent course when treatment was minimized in response to a request or demand of this sort. In particular, never let a patient persuade you to skimp on the dressing.

Explain to the patient that everything possible will be done to ensure maximal recovery in minimal time, but that in the final analysis, much of the ultimate result will be directly related to his or her cooperation and willingness to rehabilitate the hand. The most successful results occur with people who never make allowances for anything but a satisfactory result. A patient who assumes that the disability is severe, no matter what its physical extent, probably will experience protracted or permanent disability. Anything you can do to set the patient on the road to a positive attitude toward rehabilitation will benefit all involved.

In the recovery phase, especially following a severe injury, the patient will have to do a lot of boring, uncomfortable, hard work to gain maximal strength and dexterity. Understanding the need to assume this responsibility early in treatment will benefit the patient greatly as recovery progresses. The patient may ask about therapy. It is wise to make no promises, but you may tell the patient that now physical and occupational therapists do specialize in hand therapy, and these hand therapists can often give great help. Just knowing that such people are available can give a patient with an injured hand a big psychologic boost.

"Cure" of an injured hand is a relative concept. Usually, the final outcome is less perfect than one had hoped for, yet far better than one had feared. Perhaps it is best to strike a note of cautious optimism regarding the extent to which "normal" function can be achieved, provided the patient lives up to his or her responsibilities.

PART TWO

Specific Problems

Whoever undertakes to hew wood for the master carpenter rarely escapes injuring his own hands.

LAO TZU
CHINESE PHILOSOPHER
CA. 600 B.C.

6

Wounds, Lacerations and Foreign Bodies

THE common denominator of most of the lesions discussed in this book is a traumatic skin opening—a wound or laceration. The word laceration implies a clean, incisive type of opening, while wound conjures up a vision of a more mangled rent in the skin. However, the terms overlap somewhat and are used interchangeably in this and subsequent chapters.

With any wound the goal of treatment is to achieve solid closure as soon as possible. The quickest and best way to do this may not always be readily apparent. Just as the shortest distance between two points may not always be a straight line, the route to successful wound closure may not be direct suture. It does little good to close a wound under such tension that necrosis, slough, and possibly infection follow. In such a situation, open treatment followed by skin grafting would be far more appropriate.

Wound Classification

Every hand laceration or wound may be classified in two ways: as tidy or untidy, simple or complex.

TIDY WOUNDS

As the term implies, tidy wounds are neat, clean, almost surgical skin openings. The laceration may be long or short and may or may not involve deeper structures, but it lacks extensive disruption and maceration of skin or subcutaneous tissue (Fig. 6-1).

UNTIDY WOUNDS

These lacerations or wounds are characterized by torn, jagged skin edges with subcutaneous disruption. It may be difficult to determine the viability of some shreds of skin. Often foreign material is present in such wounds, and may even be ground into the tissues (Fig. 6-2).

SIMPLE WOUNDS

An injury in which only the skin and subcutaneous tissue are damaged, and in which skin loss is confined to less than 1 cm.^{2} is considered a simple wound. Such wounds may be either tidy, as in Figure 6-1, or untidy, as in Figure 6-2.

COMPLEX WOUNDS

An injury in which underlying structures such as nerves or tendons have been damaged, or in which the loss of skin is greater than 1 cm.^{2} is considered a complex wound. The size limitation regarding skin loss is somewhat arbitrary, but is based

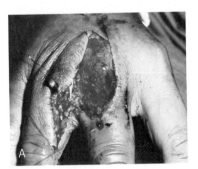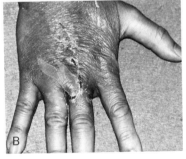

FIG. 6-1. (A) This is a large but simple, tidy wound because there is no substance loss and no injury to underlying structures. (B) The same patient three weeks after injury and repair.

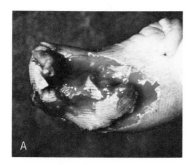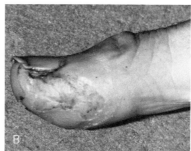

FIG. 6-2. *(A) This patient was using a power saw and sustained this simple, untidy wound. (B) The same patient 2½ weeks later.*

on the fact that defects smaller than this heal rather rapidly by epithelialization, while larger defects usually require a skin graft for expeditious closure. Occasionally large wounds may be left to heal secondarily, and small wounds treated with grafting.

Complex wounds may be tidy or untidy. Figure 6-3 gives an example of a straightforward complex wound; many of the injuries discussed in the remainder of this book are examples of complex wounds. Chapter 12 is devoted entirely to complex injuries in which there is multiple-system damage.

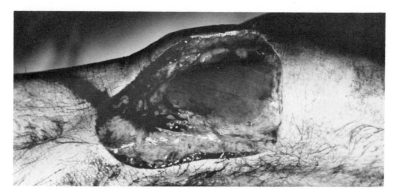

FIG. 6-3. *This young man was using a ham skinner when it skinned him. An extensive full thickness loss on the ulnar side of the hand-wrist junction is obvious. The wound is tidy but complex because of the extent of the skin loss.*

With most wounds, the correct classification according to these categories and the requisite treatment are obvious. Occasionally a wound may seem more or less difficult than it actually is until one classifies it, and then the problem (or lack of same) becomes much more apparent.

Treatment of Lacerations

GENERAL PRINCIPLES

Always use a tourniquet to render the field bloodless and use anesthesia. If local infiltration anesthesia is used, I recommend that the solution be introduced through the wound rather than through the intact skin. In general, block anesthesia is preferable.

Careful handling of the tissues with fine instruments is the first step in repair. Skin is precious; it must be debrided conservatively and handled gently. An often neglected tissue is the subcutaneous fat. This is relatively avascular, does not regenerate, and provides essential padding between the skin and underlying structures. It should be handled with care and preserved with diligence.

Dead space is difficult to define with precision but obvious when observed in vivo; it has been likened to a hot dog bun from which the hot dog has been removed. It is an empty closed space in living tissue created either by the wounding agent or by the surgeon. If it cannot be obliterated surgically, it should be left open or drained with a small Penrose drain (see Fig. 6-1). The danger of neglecting dead space is that of providing a congenial milieu for pathogens, since the space will fill with tissue fluid which is an ideal culture medium.

TECHNIQUES OF CLOSURE

The instruments and suture materials outlined in Part I should be used. No matter what type of suture is chosen, it should cause the skin edges to be slightly everted. The ideal suture brings the cut edges of the skin together exactly, but this is difficult to achieve in practice and slight eversion causes almost the same

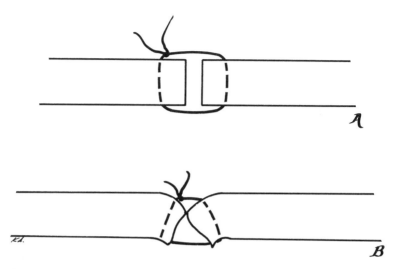

FIG. 6-4. *The suture should be pulled tight enough to approximate the skin edges (A) but not so tight that it inverts them (B).*

effect. Inversion of skin edges delays healing, as do gaps between skin edges. A well-placed simple suture tied with the right amount of tension will accomplish the goal nicely. Figure 6-4 shows the right and wrong way to put in a simple suture. Knots should always be square and set down flat. If the first throw of the knot is doubled (the so-called surgeon's knot), there is less chance of the knot slipping before the second, cinching throw is put down. A vertical mattress suture (Fig. 6-5) causes the skin edges to evert nicely. The disadvantage of this type of suture is that the suture material may become buried and difficult to remove.

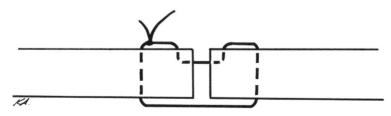

FIG. 6-5. *The vertical mattress suture is useful to evert the skin edges.*

In wounds with angular components the corner stitch may be useful. In this stitch the needle is passed through the full thickness of the skin of the nonflap side near the angle of the wound. It is then used to pick up the subcuticular layer of the flap at its angle (Fig. 6-6A). Finally, the needle is passed through the nonflap side of the wound on the other side of the angle (Fig. 6-6B). This suture neatly snugs the edge of the flap down to its proper position, properly everted (Fig. 6-6C).

In long wounds a running suture is useful, such as the running horizontal mattress suture. This is started as a simple stitch and then continued along the wound (see Fig. 6-7). If the wound to be sutured is long, it is best to put a simple suture after every four or five mattress sutures to make removal easier.

Sometimes closure of an injury is not possible at the time of primary treatment. Closure under tension is fraught with secondary problems and should be avoided. Skin grafts or flaps are often necessary for such wounds, either primarily or as delayed procedures. Urgent closure of wounds is rarely necessary if careful surgical technique is maintained and sterile dressings are applied.

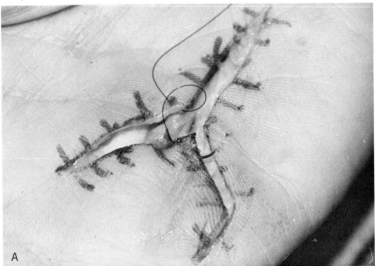

A

FIG. 6-6. (A) The first two "bites" of a corner stitch. (Continued on facing page.)

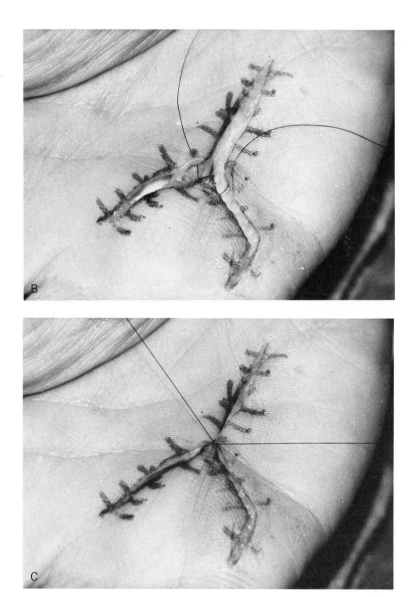

(FIG. 6-6 Cont'd.)   (B) *The corner stitch completed. (C) The corner stitch tied.*

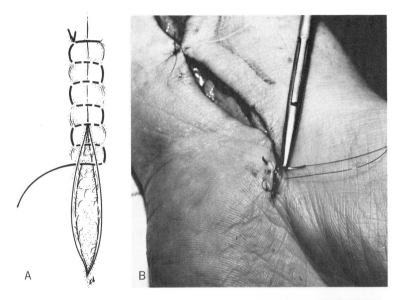

A   B

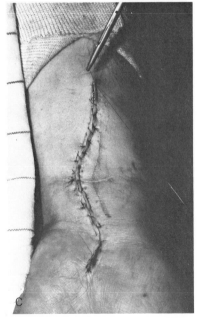

FIG. 6-7. (A) *Diagram of a running horizontal mattress suture. (B) This long wound has been pulled together with a vertical mattress suture in the midportion. A running horizontal mattress suture has been started at one end. (C) The running horizontal mattress stitch is concluded. Intermittent simple stitches have been placed to make suture removal easier.*

Although referral is often necessary in these cases, the next chapter will demonstrate that it is not always mandatory.

TIDY WOUNDS

A simple, tidy laceration is closed by suturing. A frequently asked question is whether or not one should close wounds in layers. When handling wounds in the forearm, wrist, or hand, the answer is generally no. The fascia is multilayered or ill-defined in many places, and the structures beneath function well without fascia. To close fascia in areas where it is well defined, such as the volar forearm, is to invite initiation of Volkmann's ischemic contracture (please refer to Chapter 12 for more details). In the forearm, small fascial rents should be enlarged to avoid the development of any possible constriction of underlying structures.

A tidy complex wound does not necessarily require immediate referral, as will be outlined in subsequent chapters. It does mean that the injury to deep structures must be recognized and appropriately managed. A simple example is a lacerated vessel, which should be identified, clamped precisely, and ligated or cauterized. Few outpatient departments or offices have a cautery readily available, and therefore, ligation with 6-0 nylon or a similar material is done. Blind clamping in bleeding wounds often leads to iatrogenic injury, especially to digital nerves; the use of a tourniquet is manadatory.

A special example of a tidy simple wound is a flap laceration, which may be based either proximally or distally. In general, proximally based flaps have a better circulation and a better chance of survival than distally based flaps. If there seems any possibility of flap survival, tacking the flap down with a few sutures and following the patient closely is the wisest course. One can always amputate the flap and supply a skin graft if necessary, but it is better to give nature a chance at repair first.

UNTIDY WOUNDS

Untidy wounds are usually, but not always, obvious. Occasionally one is surprised to see tissue maceration and foreign debris in a wound that appears clean at the surface. Loose dirt and debris should be removed manually and by irrigation. Irrigation should be adequate but not excessive—there seems little necessity to turn the emergency department into a bathhouse. If dirt is ground into tissue that otherwise appears viable, the tissue should be spared. Remember that the hand has a rich circulation, and tissue that is not severely traumatized by the wounding agent or the surgeon usually heals well. In this regard, vigorously scrubbing wounds is ill-advised. Scrubbing is excessively traumatic and will lead to swelling and compromise of circulation.

Untidy complex wounds usually need early referral and this decision is seldom difficult to make. The urgency of referral depends on the degree of tissue destruction, which deep structures are involved, and the extent of skin loss.

Foreign Bodies

The surgical removal of foreign bodies from the hand and forearm varies in degree of difficulty from absurdly easy to totally impossible. All kinds of small objects and particles may pierce the skin and penetrate the hand, wrist, or forearm to varying depths.

In obtaining the history several questions must be answered. What type of material is the foreign body? Organic materials, especially certain types of wood, have a potential for causing tissue reaction (Fig. 6-8) that glass or metal (Fig. 6-9) do not have, and therefore removal is more urgent. How long has the foreign body been present? If the injury is not acute, referral is the wisest course. Is the foreign body symptomatic? Often the patient's primary concern is more mental than physical (especially about "migration" of the foreign body); the actual physical symptoms may be minimal or nonexistent.

A careful history and physical examination give much information regarding direction of penetration, depth of penetration, and damage to underlying structures. Unless the foreign body is readily apparent, a roentgenogram should be obtained. Even if one suspects that the object is not radiopaque, a shadow may appear that could be helpful. Xerograms sometimes show an

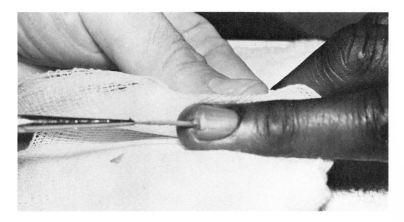

FIG. 6-8. *A large wooden splinter is removed from beneath a nail after notching the distal nail margin. A digital block should be administered before doing this.*

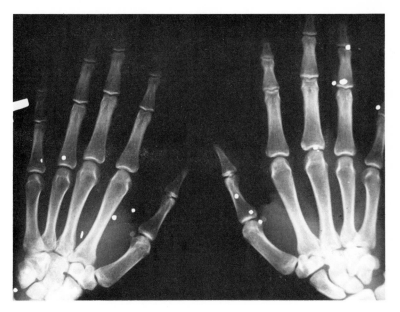

FIG. 6-9. *These shotgun pellets are fairly innocuous and can be removed if and when they come to skin level.*

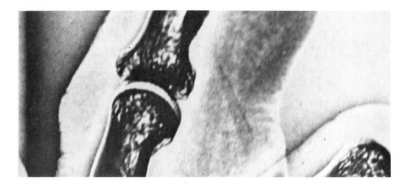

FIG. 6-10. *This xerogram clearly shows a foreign body in the soft tissue. It was a large wooden splinter.*

otherwise nonradiopaque foreign body (Fig. 6-10). Several views are mandatory and metal skin markers may be helpful in localizing the object. Of course, it is essential that the roentgenograms be displayed on a viewer while one is exploring for the foreign body. If an image intensifier is available, it should be used—this tool infinitely simplifies the location and removal of a radiopaque foreign body.

The biggest error made in searching for a foreign body is unrealistic persistence. Before commencing the search, which is always done with anesthesia and tourniquet, the patient should be warned that a timed, limited search will be conducted and if no foreign body is found, the search will be terminated. The search should last ten minutes. If it is unsuccessful, the wound is closed and the patient is referred to a consultant. In comparison to immediate retrieval of the foreign body this is an inconvenience to the patient in terms of time and expense. However, it is in persistent rummaging through tissue that nerves are cut iatrogenically and infection commenced. It is better to inconvenience the patient briefly than to injure the hand.

REFERENCES

1. McGregor, I.: Fundamental Techniques of Plastic Surgery. 8th ed. London, Churchill Livingstone, 1975.

7

Injuries to the Fingerpad, Nail and Nailbed

J UST as the prow of a ship is the section that most often strikes
a submerged object, so the tip of the finger is the part that is
most often smashed or lacerated. A wound of the distal
finger may be very painful. Unless it heals rapidly, it is inconvenient and, for many occupations, disabling.

Fingerpad Injuries

These injuries may be either tidy or untidy. The wound may be
complex by virtue of nerve, tendon, or bone injury, or because of
significant loss of skin. If the wound is simple, follow the principles of treatment outlined in Chapter 7. Nerve, tendon, or bone
injuries are discussed in their respective chapters. In general,
injuries to these tissues occur less frequently and are less important than the problem of skin loss.

THE NORMAL FINGERPAD

The fingerpad runs from the DIP flexion crease to the distal
nail margin. Laterally it extends to the dorsal skin corresponding
approximately to a line joining the dorsal part of the DIP flexion
crease and the proximal nail margin. The skin is tethered at these
margins by fascial bands, which are interspersed throughout the
pad in the subcutaneous fat. Because of these fascial strands, the

93

pad is soft and resilient without being mushy or unable to retain its shape. The skin of the pad is thick and resistant to trauma. The pad is highly sensible owing to a rich supply of nerve endings from the two volar digital nerves. These nerves arborize into their fine terminal branches near the DIP level. The blood supply from the two digital arteries is also excellent.

SKIN LOSS

Part or all of the pad may be sliced or torn away by a variety of injuries. There are five possible methods to treat the loss of skin caused by these injuries:

1. creeping epithelialization
2. a split-thickness skin graft
3. a full-thickness skin graft
4. local advancement flaps
5. a distant pedicle flap.

Creeping epithelialization is an excellent method if the wound is small (Fig. 7-1). As suggested in Chapter 6, 1 cm.^{2} should be regarded the largest area of skin loss treatable by this method. Sometimes it may be useful to graft wounds smaller than this to accelerate the healing process.

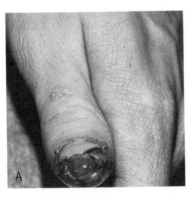 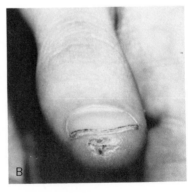

FIG. 7-1. (A) *This young man sustained a small avulsion of his left distal thumb pad, shown here four days after injury. (B) Twenty-six days after injury, excellent healing has taken place by creeping epithelialization.*

In the acute situation, the use of split-thickness skin grafts is the preferred method of treating larger injuries (more than 1 cm.^{2}). A thin split-thickness graft serves as a biologic dressing to promote rapid healing. As healing progresses, considerable shrinkage occurs and the size of the original wound is reduced by 50% or more. Because pad skin is tethered at the edges, this contracture does not produce a flexion contracture across a joint, but causes the normal pad skin to stretch. The same phenomenon occurs in wound epithelialization, but without the rapid initial healing that characterizes split-thickness grafting. The ultimate character of the skin graft is usually good. The technique of split thickness skin grafting appears on pages 96–99.

Full-thickness skin grafting is more time-consuming to execute than the split-thickness skin graft because the graft must be sutured in place. It shrinks little or none on healing and thus the size of the defect does not lessen appreciably. The ultimate outcome of this type of graft is often not much better than that with the split-thickness graft. The full-thickness graft is an excellent and useful technique in other areas of the hand, but it is seldom the graft of choice for the fingerpad in the acute situation.

There are two basic types of local advancement flaps with many modifications. Normal skin proximal to the wound is incised along two lateral margins in a V-shape, creating a triangle, with the third side being the wound margin. This flap is then totally freed from all dermal connections, leaving only a subcutaneous attachment. It may then be advanced to cover the wound partly or totally. Originally Kutler described this type of flap, which consisted of two flaps taken from either side of the finger and advanced over the defect (Fig. 7-2). The defect created by advancement of the flaps is sutured directly. Atasoy and co-workers described a flap created from volar skin that is similar in concept (Fig. 7-3). These flaps are useful in selected situations, but their execution is more difficult than the diagrams might lead one to believe. The flaps are also fairly slow to heal. An indication for a flap advancement procedure would be a deep gouging defect with large amounts of pad skin remaining. Please be wary of doing these procedures without having first seen them performed by an experienced operator.

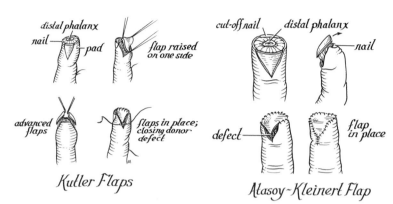

FIG. 7-2.   *Diagrams showing the techniques of the Kutler flap and the Atasoy-Kleinert flap operations. Despite the appearance of simplicity, they are complicated procedures.*

Distant pedicle flaps are the fifth method for fingerpad coverage. These may be taken from another finger, the palm, or a more distant site. In my opinion they have virtually no place in the acute treatment of fingerpad injuries. In the acute situation it is difficult to assess accurately the wound contamination, the potential for stiffness if the finger is rigidly held for the two to three weeks for a pedicle to "set," and the patient's psychologic ability to tolerate this treatment. If the pedicle does not succeed, far more harm may result than that inflicted by the original injury. These distant flaps have a place in treatment as secondary procedures, but seldom as primary procedures.

METHOD OF SPLIT-THICKNESS SKIN GRAFTING

The advantages of thin split-thickness skin grafts have already been stated. They cover denuded soft tissue easily, and in fingertip injuries they also take on bone and tendon because these tissues are surrounded by well-vascularized soft tissues. Almost always some paratenon, which has vascular supply, remains on the tendon. Injured bones in the distal phalanx tend to reveal a surface of well-vascularized cancellous bone. Bone spicules must be smoothed off with a small rongeur prior to application of a graft.

Although any convenient donor site may be used, the ipsilateral low volar forearm in a hairless area is ideal. Many experienced hand surgeons, especially those whose orientation is in plastic surgery, take exception to this choice of donor site because it might leave an unsightly scar on the forearm. I have never found this to be a problem in the large number of cases I have done personally. If the graft is properly taken and is quite thin, the resulting scar on the forearm becomes nearly invisible after a few months. Alternative sites for graft harvest include the medial upper arm or the buttock. The obvious advantage of using the forearm as a donor site is that it already lies within the field of the tourniquet.

The patient with the injured fingertip is put on the treatment table with the hand supported, a tourniquet in place (Fig. 7-3), and the digit as well as an appropriate forearm patch of skin anesthetized.

The steps of this procedure are shown in Figure 7-4. After the two areas have been blocked anesthetically and the hand and

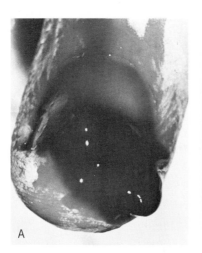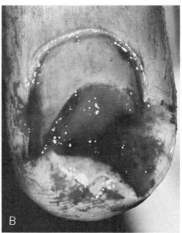

FIG. 7-3. *This patient gouged out a portion of his nail, nailbed, and fingerpad while slicing onions. (A) Appearance of the wound before the tourniquet was applied to the arm. (B) The effectiveness of the tourniquet in providing a clear, bloodless field is apparent.*

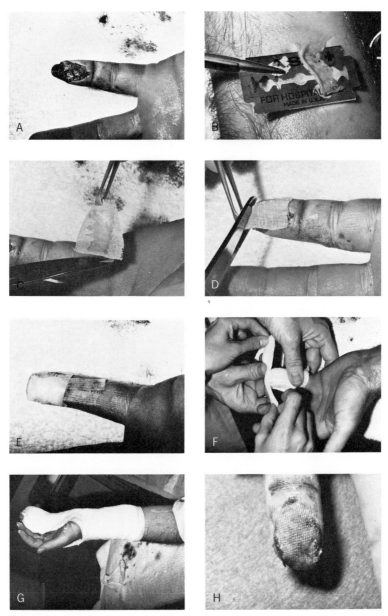

Fɪɢ. 7-4.   *(Caption on facing page.)*

forearm prepared for surgery, cut a piece of nonadherent gauze (such as Xeroform), approximately to the size of the defect to be grafted. Cut four to six thicknesses of plain gauze a little larger than this. Then elevate the arm for one minute and inflate the tourniquet to about 250 mm. of Hg. Use your nondominant hand wrapped around the patient's forearm to make the donor site taut. Holding a double-edged razor blade in a straight clamp, take the skin graft with a continuous to-and-fro motion while slowly advancing the blade. If you can read the writing on the razor blade through the skin graft, the thickness is just right. Then lay the skin on the precut piece of nonadherent gauze, with the outside layer against the gauze. It may be necessary to take a second piece of skin to get enough to cover the defect. Take enough skin to cover the defect entirely. Dress the donor site with nonadherent gauze, a wet 2 × 2 gauze, and a piece of foam sponge such as Reston.

Remove the clots on the wound by brushing them away with wet gauze or irrigation. Removal of bone spicules and debridement should be done if not performed previously. Paint the finger with tincture of benzoin, almost up to the wound edges. Lay the graft-on-gauze on the defect and cover with a sopping wet precut gauze. As soon as the benzoin is "tacky," carefully apply a ¼-inch (6.3-mm.) × 4-inch (10-cm.) porous adhesive paper strip so that the graft is not dislodged. Apply subsequent paper strips with a bit more compressive force. Ultimately, a cocoon-like effect is achieved. Further dress the finger with a 2 × 2 gauze and 1-inch (2.5-cm.) elastic gauze bandage. Incorporating an adjacent finger in the dressing is a common practice, but a thumb may be dressed alone. Then release the tourniquet. With practice, tourni-

---

Fig. 7-4. *(A) A 29-year-old man lost most of the pad of his left little finger. The wound is shown after the tourniquet was inflated. (B) The technique of taking a graft. You should be able to read the writing on the razor blade through the graft. (C) The graft is placed outside down on a piece of nonadherent gauze (Xeroform). (D) Graft and nonadherent gauze are applied to the defect. (E) A "cocoon" is built with porous adhesive paper strips (Steri-Strips). (F) Foam sponge strips (Reston) may be added over the gauze on the finger dressing. (G) Plaster cast showing the best way to dress this type of injury. (H) Usually within seven to ten days adherence of the graft is excellent.*

quet time need be no more than 10 minutes. Construction of an appropriate plaster shell completes the dressing. The usual support measures and follow-up arrangements are made.

The cast is removed seven to ten days after grafting. Almost always, the patient and the surgeon are rewarded with a wound that has closed by a primary take of the graft. Care should be exercised at the first dressing change to avoid dislodging the graft. If fine scissors are used to cut the porous adhesive paper strips next to the nonadherent-gauze bolus, and if the gauze bolus is teased away from the graft, no harm will be done. Expose the donor site totally. The finger may now be dressed with a loosely applied small adhesive bandage and a finger guard. Cover the donor site with a similar adhesive bandage, also loosely applied. Instruct the patient to change these dressings at home, allowing some "open" time for the healing wounds to dry out completely. From this point on, the injured part can be used progressively while exercising reasonable caution. It is most instructive to record the wound area in millimeters at the time of injury, at the first dressing change, and subsequently thereafter to determine how much shrinkage has actually occurred (Fig. 7-5).

The reader may wonder why sutures are not used to hold the graft down and then tied over a bolus of wet cotton. This is a time-honored and practical technique used with thick split-thickness or full-thickness grafts. In my opinion it is far too time-consuming and totally unnecessary in the acute treatment of

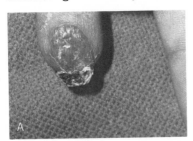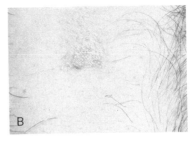

FIG. 7-5. *Five weeks after grafting. (A) The graft has noticeably shrunk in size; compare with Fig. 7-4(H). Such contracture is an advantage of the thin split-thickness graft. (B) The scar at the donor site fades just as soon, as demonstrated here.*

fingerpad injuries. Under these circumstances, the whole objective is to achieve early rapid healing with a biologic dressing.

If the coverage provided by the split-thickness graft proves unsatisfactory for the patient's ultimate needs, one may resort to another technique to provide thicker coverage, as by cross-finger, thenar, cross-arm, or other distant pedicle flaps. In the case of the thumb, one might even consider performing a neurovascular island pedicle flap. The point is that these procedures may be planned in advance, permitting maximal patient comprehension and consent, and be executed electively under conditions that favor an optimal result. None of these conditions prevails in the acute situation.

Split-thickness skin grafts have been used successfully for repair of fingerpad injuries in patients as young as two years and as old as 80. Interestingly, the need or desire for revisionary procedures following split-thickness skin grafting has been infrequent. Moreover, some patients who have requested further procedures, such as a flap procedure, have not been satisfied despite the fact that technically satisfactory results were obtained with these procedures of greater magnitude. Such patients must come to the realization that a completely normal finger cannot be restored, and that their lives must proceed with whatever results can be reasonably obtained.

Nail and Nailbed Injuries

These injuries run the gamut from a simple subungual hematoma to a complex nail avulsion with a torn nailbed and displaced fracture of the distal phalanx. Injuries at this level, even those that involve a distal phalangeal fracture, almost never result in a mallet deformity. With these injuries especially, early correct treatment can save the patient a lot of misery.

THE NORMAL NAIL APPARATUS

As described in Chapter 1 (see especially Fig. 1-7), the nail emanates from a sulcus on the dorsal finger. That part of the nail that is buried, one-quarter to one-third of its total length, has germinal matrix on both surfaces. The visible part of the nail has nongerminal or sterile matrix beneath it. Only nail matrix separates the nail from the distal phalanx. The nail will not grow unless germinal matrix is present, nor will it adhere unless sterile matrix is present. The normal skin fold at the base of the nail is called the eponychium or eponychial fold.

SUBUNGUAL HEMATOMA

This is the most common nail injury; it is caused by compression or a sharp direct blow (Fig. 7-6). As blood fills the potential space between nail and nailbed, the pressure exerted on sensitive nerve endings is intense and painful. Releasing the hematoma by puncturing the nail affords great relief of pain. This may be accomplished by penetration with a red-hot paper clip, although occasionally the heat generated with this treatment will seal the hole. Battery-powered drills are commercially available to do the job, but they seem unnecessarily expensive. An excellent method is to anesthetize the finger and to puncture the nail about three or four times with a no. 18 needle. Zinc oxide dressings are ideal for these injuries, because in most cases they keep the holes open and draining.

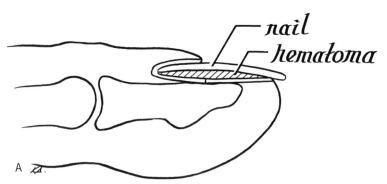

FIG. 7-6. (A) A schematic view of a subungual hematoma. (Continued on p. 103.)

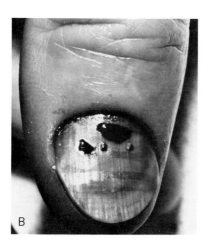

FIG. 7-6.   *(B) A typical subungual hematoma being drained through several holes made in the nail.*

B

THE AVULSED NAIL

Avulsion of a nail at its base by a sharp blow delivered to the distal end is a common injury. The nail is literally levered out of its basal attachment, and the base comes to lie on the eponychium (Figs. 7-7, 7-8A). The injury may consist only of the avulsed nail, but in many instances the underlying nail matrix has been injured as well (Fig. 7-8B). Because the nail is no longer connected with the germinal matrix, a new nail must grow out of this germinal matrix. There is a widespread but erroneous belief that the avulsed nail, if left in place, will act as a "splint" for the new nail

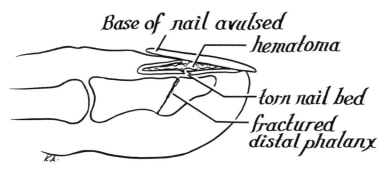

FIG. 7-7.   *Avulsion of the nail.*

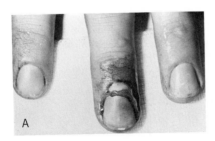
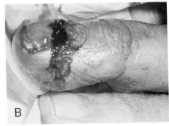

FIG. 7-8.   (A) *Typical appearance of a nail avulsed at the base.* (B) *Usually, after removing the avulsed nail, one can clearly see injuries to the sterile matrix, which has been torn and displaced in this case.*

while it is growing into place. Leaving the avulsed nail in place hides underlying injury to the nailbed and may prolong or even prevent proper healing. The inert nail acts as a foreign body, irritating the sensitive nailfold and nailbed; furthermore, it creates

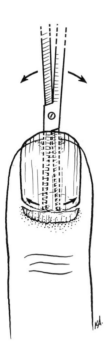

dead space that provides an excellent environment for infection. If the old nail, or even part of it, is left in place, it will mechanically interfere with the growth of the new nail. Thus it should be removed, even if it remains attached to the sterile matrix (see Fig. 7-9). Once the injured matrix is uncovered, sutured, and allowed to heal, it loses its sensitivity rapidly (Fig. 7-10). If no injury has occurred to the germinal matrix, a new nail will have grown in place in about three to four months.

FIG. 7-9.   *Technique for removing an avulsed nail. Introducing the clamp at the distal end of the nail where it is still attached avoids stressing the injured nailbed.*

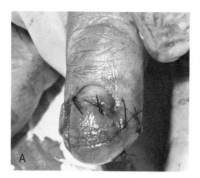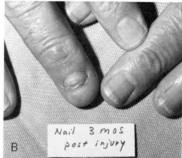

FIG. 7-10. (A) *The matrix may be sutured with either nylon or an absorbable suture. (B) Three months after injury the nailbed is dry and nontender and the new nail is advancing.*

Combined Injury

An injury to the distal finger may involve pad, nail, nailbed, and the distal phalanx itself. The distal phalanx is important only because it provides pain-free support to the soft tissue structures; exact apposition of bony ends in a fracture is not mandatory to achieve this end. If the soft tissues are carefully aligned and sutured, the bone usually comes into a satisfactory position. Fracture fixation, which may be required occasionally, is discussed in Chapter 11.

In this type of injury the nailbed may be so shattered that only remnants of it remain. Any section of germinal matrix that does remain is capable of producing pieces of nail or so-called nail horns. These are unsightly and annoying because they constantly snag on objects (Fig. 7-11). Sometimes several surgical procedures are required to eliminate all of them. With combined injuries, the goal of treatment is to obtain early healing without a painful scar. Often secondary procedures are required, and these have been discussed in the first part of this chapter.

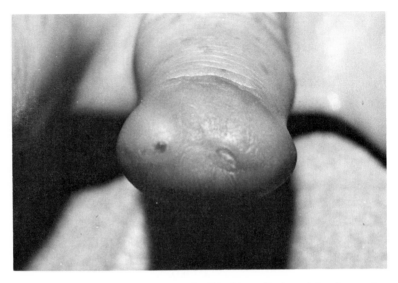

FIG. 7-11. *Two nail horns appear in this finger that sustained amputa-tion of most of the distal phalanx some months previously.*

REFERENCES

FINGERPAD INJURIES

1. Kilgore, E. S. Jr., and Newmeyer, W. L.: Fingertip injuries (Trauma Rounds). West. J. Med., *122:*521–525, 1975.

2. Newmeyer, W. L., and Kilgore, E. S., Jr.: Fingertip injuries: a simple, effective method of treatment. J. Trauma, *14:*58–64, 1974.

3. Atasoy, E., et al: Reconstruction of the amputated fingertip with a triangular volar flap. J. Bone Joint Surg., *52A:*921–926, 1970.

4. Kutler, W: A new method for fingertip amputation. JAMA, *133:*29–30, 1947.

NAIL AND NAILBED INJURIES

5. Newmeyer, W. L., and Kilgore, E. S., Jr: Common Injuries of the Fingernail and Nailbed. Am. Family Phys., *16:*93–95, 1977.

8

Infections of the Hand

MINOR infections of the hand, especially of the digits, are fairly common. Minor implies that they do not necessitate hospitalization of the patient and that the pathologic process usually subsides in two to three days with proper treatment. However, even a minor infection may create a major problem for the patient in activities of daily living both at home and work. Fortunately, major infections that require hospitalization are fairly uncommon today. An exception to this last statement is the population of drug addicts. Severe, devastating infections that often necessitate prolonged hospitalization and not infrequently lead to loss of digits or hands are alarmingly common in this pathetic group of people.

Pathogenesis

With few exceptions, infection follows some type of penetrating trauma. The trauma may have been trivial and even forgotten by the patient by the time the infection becomes clinically apparent. Blood-borne infections are so uncommon that they are medical curiosities, although one should keep gonococcal arthritis in mind as a possible diagnosis for a "hot" joint.

To establish an infection, penetration must be compounded by a certain degree of tissue congestion and the introduction of some pathogen. Often self-neglect, iatrogenic neglect, or ill-advised therapy plays a significant role in propagating infection. Self-neglect is a problem particularly associated with people who have lost full conscious control of their bodies by reason of drugs, age, or disease. (See Fig. 8-1).

Any penetration into tissue is followed by some local increase in extracellular fluid. This extravasation of fluid causes tissue congestion, which decreases the efficiency of tissue perfusion— especially venous and lymphatic return. If the process continues unchecked, the pressure within the tissue may become so great that arterial flow is cut off and death of the tissue results. In such congested tissue, pathogens can thrive and virulent microorganisms can blossom. The propagation of organisms may cause formation of an abscess, which further compresses tissue, or if no abscess forms, more extracellular fluid accumulates to cause more compression. This vicious cycle is illustrated in Figure 8-2.

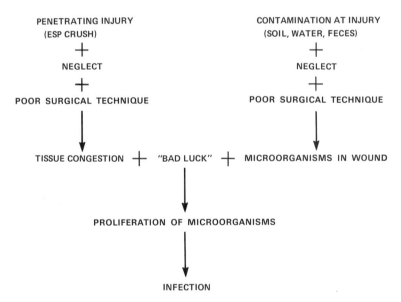

FIG. 8-1. *Blood-borne infections are not common in the hand. Many infections have a large element of self-neglect or ill-choosen or insufficient therapy in their genesis. As indicated here, "bad luck" may also play a part, and sometimes infections arise even with the most assiduous care.*

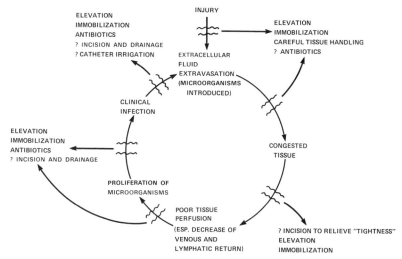

FIG. 8-2.   *This schematic representation of the mechanical factors of infection suggests ways to abort the impending problem in the early phases. Maintaining good tissue perfusion remains, by far, the most important single factor in preventing infection.*

Principles of Treatment

The first and most important step in treating an infection is to relieve tissue congestion, thereby restoring maximal tissue perfusion. This swelling or tissue congestion must be relieved by the most direct method appropriate to the situation. Elevation to heart level or above is obviously required, both acutely and until the infection has subsided completely.

If subcutaneous or subfascial pressure is playing a significant role, incision of the skin or fascial envelope is necessary. Surgical release of tight skin or fascia will permit both drainage of pus and alleviation of the constriction, so that the improvement in tissue perfusion becomes immediately obvious. Relief of pain is a significant additional bonus of this step.

Of course, any such cavity surgically created constitutes dead space, and it must be drained properly to permit healing to progress from below and to prevent a repetition of the same process of congestion. This may require placing a pack of iodoform gauze or a similar material in the wound. Beware of packing an abscess or any other cavity so tightly that tissue congestion recurs iatrogenically. In many instances, inserting a small soft rubber drain in the wound or just coating the wound with zinc oxide prevents adherence of the edges of the wound and sealing of the cavity.

Diagnostic Adjuncts

SPECIMEN CULTURE AND SUSCEPTIBILITY TESTING

Should one culture specimens taken from every wound? Academically, identification of microorganisms should be obtained for completeness. However, the pathogens causing the great majority of infections of the hand that require incision and drainage are obvious clinically (most often being Staphylococcus aureus), and surgical drainage is definitive treatment. More often than not, the patient is well on his way to cure by the time a culture report can be returned.

Certain infections require culture of specimens or some other test to make a definitive diagnosis; these are discussed later in this chapter. Do not overlook the gram stain of a smear taken from pus or exudate. This procedure may be especially useful in suspected gonococcal or gas gangrene infections. In every case, consider the necessity for and usefulness of such testing before automatically ordering a culture and susceptibility tests.

ROENTGENOGRAMS

Are roentgenograms of infected hands necessary? With the exception of superficial infections, roentgenograms of the hand are indicated for two reasons, especially when the infection is persistent or severe. First, the inciting penetration may have implanted a radiopaque foreign body, whose removal is necessary for cure of the infection. Secondly, one should determine whether bones or joints are involved in the infection. If this is the case, more extensive surgical and antibiotic treatment is necessary than when only soft tissues are involved.

Roentgenograms may also reveal the presence of subcutaneous air bubbles, although they are not taken specifically for this purpose. Air may have been introduced mechanically at the time of injury; more ominously, the air bubbles may originate from an anaerobic infection, the most serious of which is clostridial myonecrosis. (These infections are discussed in more detail later in this chapter.)

The Question of Antibiotics

The primary care physician must decide whether or not to administer antibiotics. Patients with severe infections or unusual infections are usually referred for hospitalization. In these cases, antibiotic therapy is necessary, but the choice is out of the hands of the primary care physician.

A large number of patients have infections of the hand that require treatment with antibiotics, and the physician must determine which antibiotic is most appropriate. However, before choosing a specific antibiotic, one must be sure that the infection has been adequately treated by surgical means (incision and drainage), and that the hand is adequately immobilized and elevated. Such a determination is based on the clinician's personal knowledge and experience.

Three large studies of hand infections which were published within the last decade closely agree about the types of organisms responsible for the infections and the efficacy of antibiotic treatment.[1,2,3] One of these studies[1] compared data obtained from the same hospital in both 1947 and 1974. The most striking finding was that most cases of infection were caused by staphylococci, most of which were susceptible to penicillin in 1947, but two-thirds of which were penicillin-resistant in 1974. This report merely confirms a widely known unhappy clinical fact.

The three studies agree that 50% to 60% of hand infections are caused by staphylococci, and that one-half to two-thirds of these cases are resistant to penicillin. Another 12% to 17% of infections are caused by beta-hemolytic and other streptococci. Of the remaining cases, 7% to 10% are due to gram-positive organisms other than those mentioned here. Gram-negative microorganisms accounted for no more than 16% of the cases in any of the studies.

Antibiotic therapy should be predicated on the physician's diagnosis of the major offending organism. If it is Staphylococcus, the chances of it being penicillin-resistant are good, and you should choose a synthetic or semisynthetic penicillin such as cloxacillin or dicloxacillin taken orally. If the patient is allergic to penicillin, the drug of choice is erythromycin. A cephalosporin may also be considered, but be aware of the possibility of an allergic cross-reaction with penicillin.

If the patient has a streptococcal infection, penicillin remains the drug of choice with erythromycin as the first alternative. Clindamycin is an effective drug against gram-positive organisms, but it may produce pseudomembranous enterocolitis. Cephalosporins are effective against streptococci except S. faecalis.

Hand infections caused by gram-negative cocci are often mixed infections and, if serious enough to require antibiotic therapy, often necessitate hospitalization of the patient because the drugs of choice are available only for intramuscular or intravenous administration. Coliforms may respond to cephalosporins, but an aminoglycoside is the first choice. Proteus may respond to ampicillin. Aerobacter infections require colistin or gentamicin. Pseudomonas is treated with gentamicin combined with carbenicillin. An excellent discussion of these drugs in relation to musculoskeletal infections has been written by Wilkowske and Hermans.[4]

Should antibiotics be administered to patients with injuries that are fresh and not infected? That is, should they be used prophylactically? This remains one of the simmering controversies in medicine today. Practically, few clinicians fail to use antibiotics if the wound has a high potential for infection, either because of the degree of tissue maceration (Fig. 8-3), or because it was incurred in a contaminated setting. In such a setting, contamination from soil, feces, or other organic materials (such as dirty needles) may have occurred. I usually administer erythromycin, cloxacillin, or an oral cephalosporin in these situations.

If antibiotics are to be used prophylactically in a noninfected injury, they must be administered as soon as possible after injury.

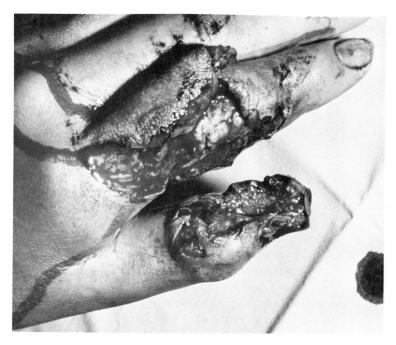

FIG. 8-3.   *This 15-year-old boy was making fireworks at home when his creation exploded prematurely. In this type of wound the use of prophylactic antibiotics may be the deciding factor in preventing infection.*

Preferably, the first dose should be administered in the emergency department or office. (A prescription that remains unfilled does little good; this is the fate of many prescriptions, especially those written at night.)

Antibiotics should never be used as a screen behind which the physician can abrogate his or her responsibility to carefully debride the wound, to handle the injured hand with utmost care and gentleness, and to properly immobilize and elevate the hand. Antibiotics are adjuncts to treatment and do not replace fundamental principles of good wound care and aftercare. Nor must the physician fail to provide adequate safeguards against the dangers of tetanus. Either tetanus immune globulin-human (Hyper-Tet) or a tetanus toxoid booster shot should be given. Tetanus toxoid, however, need not be repeated if the patient has received a primary series or a booster shot within five years. This time interval is reduced to one year if the wound is tetanus-prone (that is, if it is extensively contaminated or macerated).

If a patient is to be sent home after the initial treatment of an infection, he or she should be carefully instructed regarding signs of toxicity and to return immediately if they occur. Definite follow-up arrangements should always be made.

Specific Hand Infections

Certain infections of the hand merit specific consideration and discussion because their treatment is unique by virtue of their anatomic location, the danger they pose to hand function if they continue unchecked, or the unusual or highly virulent nature of the pathogens that are responsible for the infection.

In general, hand infections may be classified as those that involve subcuticular areas, subcutaneous space, or deep structures. The anatomy of the pad and nail gives rise to some interesting problems with infections of the distal finger. For the purposes of this discussion, simple infections are defined as those that can usually be treated in the office or emergency department, after which the patient can be sent home. Complex infections usually require hospital admission and sometimes a trip to the operating room. As the reader may surmise, the distinction between the two is not absolute.

SIMPLE INFECTIONS

The vast majority of hand infections fall into this category. Included are the paronychia, the felon, some cases of cellulitis, subcuticular abscesses, some subcutaneous abscesses, and some infected lacerations.

PARONYCHIA

This is probably the most common infection of the hand. The cross-section anatomy of the distal finger is shown in Figure 8-4.

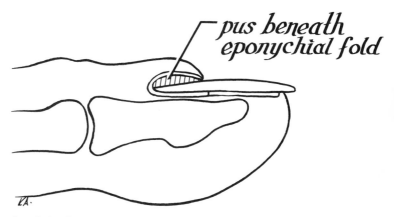

FIG. 8-4.   *A paronychia is shown schematically.*

The proximal one-quarter to one-third of the nail is tucked into a sulcus called the eponychial fold. The nail is separated from the distal phalanx and the skin fold by nail matrix, which is germinal proximal to the fold and sterile distal to it.

Infections under this nailfold may occur readily from a seemingly trivial injury. Often the infection is initiated when the patient picks or pulls at loose skin ("hangnails"). Usually an area of the eponychium becomes inflamed, following which a small abscess becomes apparent at some area (Fig. 8-5). The pus may spread

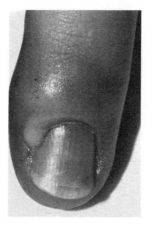

FIG. 8-5.   *Typical appearance of paronychia.*

around the entire nailfold to form a horseshoe or run-around paronychia. It may even spread under the proximal border of the nail, lifting the nail away from the nailbed to form a subungual abscess. From there the infection can dissect subcuticularly around the pad (Fig. 8-6). However, it does not penetrate beneath the dermis and remains a localized although often painful affliction.

The treatment is simple and classic: release the pus. As a first step, the digit is anesthetized and a tourniquet is used. In a simple paronychia, the eponychial fold is pushed back with the edge of a number eleven knife blade until the pus is released (Fig. 8-7A). This method is far preferable to an incision through the skin margin (Fig. 8-7B), which leaves a bridge of skin that often becomes necrotic. If the infection has spread beneath the nail, the nail should be removed. If it has spread around the pad, the superficial epidermal layers may be pulled away, leaving a fingertip that looks plucked but is quite intact (Fig. 8-8).

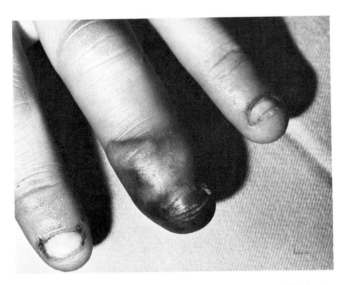

FIG. 8-6. *This patient neglected his paronychia until it had extended to the volar digit.*

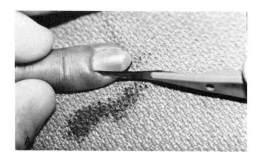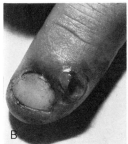

FIG. 8-7.   *(A) The correct method of draining a paronychia. (B) Draining a paronychia in this manner may permanently injure the nail margin.*

If the paronychia is treated at the cellulitic stage, rolling back the eponychium may not reveal pus. In this case, no further efforts at incision should be made.

Following release of the pus, the wound is dressed with zinc oxide, a bulky protective dressing, and usually a light splint or a plaster shell. This dressing should remain in place for two to three

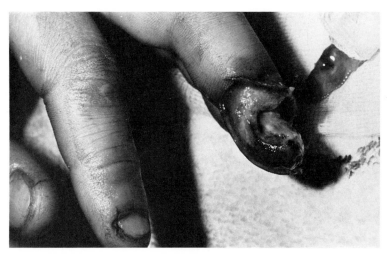

FIG. 8-8.   *Although this finger looks like a "plucked chicken," the dermal elements are intact, and except for regrowth of the nail, recovery was rapid.*

days, after which time the patient should soak the finger several times a day and dress with a small adhesive bandage.

Irritation around the eponychial fold may be caused by fungal or mixed bacterial and fungal organisms.[5] Usually this type of infection occurs in persons whose hands are chronically exposed to moisture, such as kitchen workers. An excellent treatment for this is to apply a solution composed of a few drops of 3% thymol in absolute alcohol after each exposure to moisture, and to use tolnaftate (Tinactin) cream at night. The patient should consider decreasing his or her exposure to moisture by changing jobs or using cotton-lined rubber gloves.

FELON

This is an infection of the pad of the pulp space of a digit. However, as Linscheid and Dobyns[6] stress (in an excellent monograph on hand infections for those who want information beyond the stage of emergency treatment), not every pad infection is a felon. To be a felon, the pad infection must have symptoms of severe pain and signs of tension, swelling, and marked tenderness (Figs. 8-9 and 8-10).

To appreciate why this infection should be so painful and destructive, an anatomic review is pertinent. The pad skin is stabilized at the nail margins, at the DIP flexion crease, and along

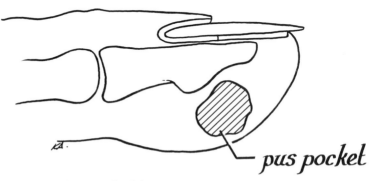

Fig. 8-9. *Diagram of a felon.*

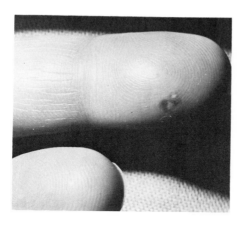

FIG. 8-10. *This patient has a typical felon that points just a bit off the midpad.*

the phalangeal border by fine fascial strands. In the center of the pad, the fascial strands are also present but less numerous. There are no true septae. Digital nerves and vessels enter the pad along each of the volar lateral borders and spread toward the center. The abscess starts somewhere in the center of the pad and is confined by the unyielding skin that is tightly tethered at the margins. The abscess is trapped, and as it enlarges, it puts intense pressure on numerous nerve endings, causing great pain.

Contrary to the continued teaching of various textbooks, the felon should be drained where it points, which is usually somewhere in the central pad (Figs. 8-11, 8-12A). Never cross the DIP

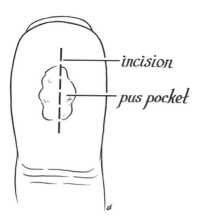

FIG. 8-11. *Felons should be drained this way—not with incisions into the side of the pad.*

—incision

—pus pocket

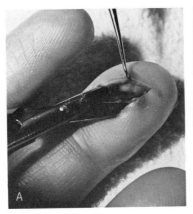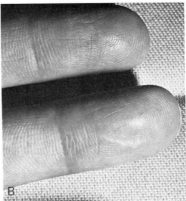

FIG. 8-12.   (A) *The felon shown in Figure 8-10 is being incised and drained. (B) The same finger after healing. There was neither pain nor tenderness.*

flexion crease directly with an incision. Assiduously avoid approaching the infection by a hockey-stick incision around the digital margin, by bilateral midaxial incisions, or by the pernicious fish-mouth incision. Reaching the infection through each of these approaches requires extensive burrowing through normal tissue, with a high probability of causing iatrogenic injury to normal neurovascular structures and injury to the fascial strands that give the pad its unique combination of resiliency and stability.[7] Following incision and drainage the wound may be kept open with a loose pack, a small rubber drain, or a coating of zinc oxide. As with other infections and injuries, a bulky dressing and a plaster shell are appropriate. The pad incision heals with a fine line that interferes little or not at all with finger function (Fig. 8-12B).

SUBEPIDERMAL ABSCESS

Small single or clustered abscesses may develop in the epidermis. These are often associated with poor hygiene. Generally, if they are unroofed with the tip of a no. 11 blade and careful hygiene is observed, no particular problems ensue.

HERPETIC LESIONS (HERPETIC WHITLOW)

This infection is often seen in medical and dental personnel. One or more painful vesicles appear on or near the fingerpad (Fig. 8-13). There may or may not be a history of herpes simplex appearing elsewhere in the body. The clinical appearance may lead one to suspect the diagnosis, which can be confirmed by the fluorescent antibody technique. Unroof the vesicle with a needle or knife blade and smear the fluid on a clear slide. Often a state laboratory will do the fluorescent antibody examination at no cost to the patient. A gram stain of the vesicular fluid will show neither polymorphonuclear cells nor bacteria.

It is most important that herpetic lesions be recognized for what they are and that extensive incision and drainage of the fingerpad not be undertaken. There is no specific treatment; the problem is self-limited.

SUBCUTANEOUS ABSCESS

These infections may run the gamut from rather small and simple lesions to large complex lesions associated with systemic toxicity. The basic treatment is incision and drainage. If the ab-

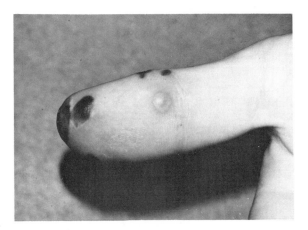

Fig. 8-13. *This is a typical vesicle of herpes simplex. Do not overtreat these lesions.*

scess occurs in an area where spread to a vital deep structure such as a tendon sheath is unlikely or not possible, definitive treatment can often be rendered in the emergency room or office with adequate anesthesia and tourniquet control. Make certain that the wound remains open and that an adequate dressing has been provided. The organism usually responsible for these infections is Staphylococcus aureus, and an appropriate antibiotic should be chosen. If the abscess is large and deep structures appear to be involved, it may be best to refer the patient for hospitalization and have drainage performed in the operating room. In practical terms, dorsal abscesses can often be managed on an outpatient basis while volar abscesses often require hospitalization. Figure 8-14 shows a typical dorsal abscess.

CELLULITIS

This is another affliction that manifests a broad spectrum in degrees of seriousness. Generally the dorsum of one or more fingers or the hand is red, tender, and swollen. There is no abscess. Ascending lymphangitis as evidenced by red streaks up the forearm may or may not be present. The causative organism is

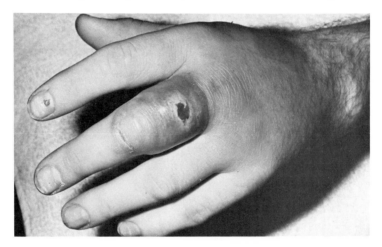

FIG. 8-14. *A young man developed this dorsal abscess after a minor laceration at work; culture Staphylococcus aureus, coagulase positive.*

usually a group A beta-hemolytic Streptococcus; treatment is with penicillin or erythromycin as a second choice. Systemic illness indicates hospital admission for intravenous antibiotic therapy. Although there is no focal point to incise, the extremity should be supported and elevated.

INFECTED WOUNDS AND LACERATIONS

As with subcutaneous abscesses and cellulitis these infections vary widely in their severity. The general mistake is to underestimate the extent of the infection and to procrastinate in treating it vigorously. If the infection occurs in a wound that you have sutured a few days previously, there is a natural reluctance to undo all the carefully placed sutures. This reluctance must be overcome and the wound or laceration opened widely. The sooner you reestablish a totally open wound—go back to ground zero so to speak—the sooner the reparative process can begin and the sooner healing will ultimately take place. A mixed flora appears in these situations, and unless the problem is small or the organism obvious, a pus sample should be obtained for gram stain, culture, and susceptibility tests. A culture for anaerobes may be indicated in some instances. Again, the importance of supporting and elevating the extremity cannot be emphasized too strongly. If the infection is severe, hospitalization may be required.

COMPLEX INFECTIONS

Certain hand infections usually owing to the nature of their location, demand hospitalization and early surgical drainage. This is not to imply that the infections discussed previously are trivial and never require this treatment; some do warrant drainage in the operating room. The injuries that follow, however, usually allow no leeway; they all demand this treatment.

SUPPURATIVE FLEXOR TENOSYNOVITIS

This infection is a true surgical emergency. When pus is trapped in a sealed flexor tendon sheath, necrosis of the flexor tendons may follow due to loss of blood supply caused by pressure. The initial trauma always is a penetrating injury, which the patient may not always be able to recall. The patient will present with a painful finger and the four signs attributed to Kanavel, a pioneer hand surgeon: (1) a red mass extends along the flexor tendon sheath; (2) the mass is very tender; (3) the finger is held rigidly in a semiflexed position; (4) passive extension of the DIP joint causes excruciating pain. This last sign is probably the most useful and the one by which a tendon sheath infection may be distinguished from a volar subcutaneous infection, which may cause the other three signs.

Occasionally, in the thumb and little finger, the flexor tendon sheath may extend to the wrist, connecting with Perona's space which lies between the pronator quadratus and the flexor tendons. Whether the infective process involves a single finger or extends to the wrist, surgical decompression is mandatory and urgent. The patient should be hospitalized and incision and drainage performed without delay.

SPACE INFECTIONS

In addition to Perona's space, infection may occur in two other potential spaces of the hand: the thenar and midpalmar spaces. According to Lampe,[8] these should more correctly be called bursa; their function is to enhance the sliding motion of the flexor tendons in relation to the underlying intrinsic muscles and metacarpals. The thenar space or bursa lies deep to the flexor tendons to the index finger and superficial to the adductor pollicis muscle belly; its lateral borders are the third metacarpal and the radial border of the hand. The midpalmar space lies deep to the flexor tendons of the long, ring, and little fingers; its lateral borders are the third metacarpal and the ulnar side of the hand.

Penetrating trauma into either space or an infection that spreads from a flexor tendon sheath may cause an abscess to form in these areas. A thenar space abscess causes swelling, redness, and tenderness in the radial midvolar palm, while these symptoms of a midpalmar abscess will appear in the ulnar midvolar palm.

Space infections are rare problems today, probably because antibiotics are commonly used early in the course of treating hand injuries. They are surgically urgent situations, and the patient should be hospitalized immediately for incision and drainage.

SEPTIC ARTHRITIS

Usually the cause of septic arthritis is obvious and straightforward. The patient gives a history of a penetrating wound and has a swollen, tender joint that is exquisitely painful on motion. If tooth penetration from a human bite is the cause, the history may have to be coaxed out of the patient (see p. 130).

If untreated, the septic arthritis will progress to destroy the articular cartilage and subchondral bone, eventually causing osteomyelitis. A roentgenogram should be obtained and the patient should be hospitalized for incision and debridement.

Gonococcal infection may cause monoarticular arthritis that is septic without a history of traumatic penetration. According to Kelly,[9] cultures of the synovial fluid usually yield gonococci in this type of arthritis. Diagnosis is confirmed by the curative response to parenteral penicillin.

OSTEOMYELITIS

Bone infection may follow a septic arthritis, and is confirmed by roentgenographic findings or radioisotope scans. Probably the most common bone infection of the hand seen today is that of the distal phalanx following a neglected or ill-treated felon or paronychia (Fig. 8-15).

If the wound can be adequately opened in the office or emergency department, it may be possible to treat a patient with osteomyelitis entirely as an outpatient. Specimens for culture must be obtained. Antibiotics must be used, probably for six to eight weeks. Pending the receipt of culture studies, antibiotic therapy should be chosen on the basis of clinical judgement regarding the type of infection or the results of a gram stain of a pus smear.

FIG. 8-15. *Osteomyelitis of the distal phalanx developed in this elderly lady after a paronychia was neglected.*

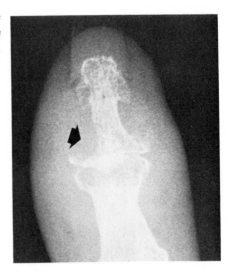

INFECTIONS IN DRUG ADDICTS

Any discussion of hand infections must mention the special problems that arise in the addict population. Hard-core addicts of long-standing do almost anything to get their drugs, and inject almost any injectable substance into themselves. Characteristically, they are ill-nourished and have poor hygiene. Generally, they exhibit chronic induration of the extremities, which indicates poor venous and lymphatic return. Last but not least, drug addicts usually neglect any infection until it is fairly advanced and very painful. All of these factors militate against early and easy resolution of the problem. Often hospitalization is required, either to ensure correct treatment that ordinarily could be done on an outpatient basis, or to treat devastating, life-threatening infections.

LIFE-THREATENING INFECTIONS

This group of infections, which are fortunately fairly uncommon, may occur in a setting of severe injury, neglect, or serious debilitation due to disease or malnutrition. It is important that these infections be recognized for the serious problems that they are (Fig. 8-16).

Clostridial myonecrosis or gas gangrene[10] is the classic life-threatening anaerobic infection, caused by one of the Clostridia organisms, usually C. perfringens. These patients are acutely ill with tachycardia and prostration, but usually have little temperature elevation. Gas in the soft tissues causes crepitation. As in other serious soft tissue infections, a gram stain of a smear is important in making the diagnosis. Wide surgical drainage with excision of dead tissue is mandatory for patient survival.

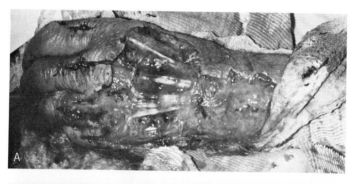

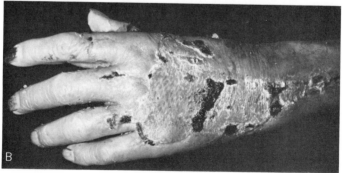

FIG. 8-16. *(A) An elderly man neglected a minor abrasion and developed an anaerobic Streptococcus infection that destroyed the skin of his dorsal hand. (B) The same patient after control of the infection and split thickness skin grafting. His hand was stiff but at least he had a hand with sensibility—far better than an amputation.*

Virulent anaerobic infections may also be caused by *anaerobic streptococci,*[11,12] although these are not as devastating as clostridial infections. Hospitalization and debridement are mandatory. A gram stain of smears will distinguish these infections from clostridial infections, and aid in the diagnosis of each. In either condition, subcutaneous gas may be seen roentgenographically. Other less devastating anaerobic infections may be caused by Escherichia coli, Klebsiella pneumoniae (Aerobacter aerogenes), and several Bacteroides species.

Necrotizing fasciitis[13] is an aggressive, devastating infection that is relatively uncommon. There is extensive necrosis of the superficial fascia with undermining of soft tissues. The patient with this disease is acutely ill with high fever. This infection may follow either traumatic or surgical wounds, but in the upper extremity it is much more likely to occur following trauma. The causative organisms are multiple and variable. As in all other serious soft tissue infections, a gram stain should guide initial antibiotic therapy pending return of culture studies. More important is that radical surgical incision and drainage beyond the limits of fascial involvement be undertaken without delay.

Meleney's synergistic gangrene is seen in wounds that are about two weeks old. There is severe pain, with central necrosis and ulceration that spread. The causative organisms are a microaerophilic nonhemolytic streptococcus and an aerobic hemolytic staphylococcus or a gram-negative rod. Again, hospitalization and surgical debridement are mandatory.

Streptococcal myositis is characterized by severe local pain in traumatic wounds. It may be due to anaerobic and aerobic streptococci. There is foul-smelling, seropurulent drainage. The skin may be tense and discolored. This infection must be differentiated from clostridial myonecrosis, and this is done by gram stain and culture. Treatment is by incision and drainage and administration of parenteral penicillin.

Other severe soft tissue infections are uncommon or not seen in the upper extremity; see the papers by Baxter[14] and by Oill et al.[15] for complete discussions. These conditions overlap in terms of the causative bacteria and other factors.

The seriousness of soft tissue infections must not be underestimated. If a patient with a soft tissue infection that looks serious also has systemic toxicity, the general course of action is to hospitalize the patient, establish a diagnosis by gram stain and culture, and in most cases perform an incision and drainage in the operating room; moreover, be prepared to support a very sick person.

Unusual Infections

Some infections of the hand are caused by uncommon pathogens. A few of the more frequent are discussed here, but this list is far from complete. To some extent the type and incidence of unusual infections depend on the climate and other local factors. Be aware of any unusual infections indigenous to your particular area that may provide a diagnosis for infections that cannot be readily identified. As a general rule these unusual infections do not demand urgent surgical measures, but eventually biopsy or special culture studies are needed for their diagnosis.

Mycobacterial infections may be either tubercular or non-tubercular. A patient with tuberculosis of the hand or wrist usually has or has had pulmonary tuberculosis. A patient with a non-tubercular mycobacterial infection invariably has contracted it from soil or water. These infections are generally insidious in onset and their diagnosis is difficult until one considers the possibility of mycobacteria. Biopsy and culture are diagnostic.[16]

A relatively uncommon group of infections are those due to *fungi*. According to Linscheid and Dobyns[6] the most common fungal infections of the hand are sporotrichosis and candidiasis.

Sporotrichosis is a fungal infection caused by Sporothrix schenckii. Infection occurs from contact with soil. A red ulcerating lesion develops at the site of injury and proximal secondary lesions may appear. Pain is minimal. Diagnosis is obtained by culture of the organism; treatment is with potassium iodide.[17]

Candida albicans is the cause of candidiasis, which is often involved at least partially as a cause of chronic paronychia. Diagnosis is obtained by examining scrapings taken from the eponychial fold. The treatment is discussed under paronychia.

Bites and Stings

These problems are fairly common, especially human bites and dog bites. The incidence of snake, spider, and insect bites may be high in some areas. A related problem is that of marine animal bites and stings, but space and lack of general applicability dictate no discussion of this topic here.

HUMAN BITES

Possibly comprising the majority of human bite wounds are tooth puncture wounds, which are bites by extrapolation only. The usual mechanism is a closed fist brought up against an opponent's upper incisors. Penetration usually occurs in the region of the dorsal MCP joint and perhaps into the joint. When the fist is opened, the line of puncture is staggered rather than straight, and the closed wound has foreign material from the mouth trapped in its depth. This may lead directly to creation of a septic joint.

Infections due to human bites usually have a mixed flora, including aerobes and anaerobes. Mann and co-workers[18] found Streptococcus the single most frequent organism, with Staphylococcus aureus the second most common. As might be expected, in over 40% of these cases the organisms were resistant to penicillin G.

The treatment of a human bite includes surgically opening the wound with debridement and copious irrigation. A gram stain and culture should be obtained. A roentgenogram may be helpful to identify bone or joint pathology. Unless it is a trivial wound initial antibiotic therapy should include a semisynthetic penicillin and gentamicin. The foregoing makes it obvious that hospitalization is often necessary (Fig. 8-17).

ANIMAL BITES

Most often these are caused by domestic dogs and cats. Pasteurella multocida is often isolated from these wounds; it is penicillin-sensitive. These wounds should be carefully debrided, irrigated, and left open or drained. Particularly with a large wound

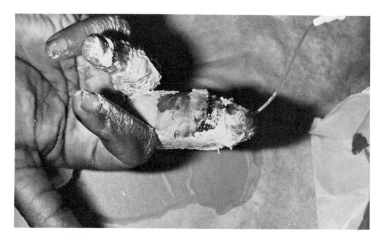

FIG. 8-17. *This young man was bitten by another man at the PIP joint. The finger is seen here in the midst of treatment, covered with zinc oxide and with an irrigation catheter protruding. He kept his finger, but the PIP joint became ankylosed. Human bites can give rise to vicious infections.*

from a dog bite, it may be necessary to do at least a partial closure to preserve viability of the skin flaps. Rabies is a threat occasionally with domestic animals, but more often with wild animals. Local public health departments have detailed protocols regarding rabies detection and management, and animal bites should be reported for this reason.

Cat scratches may result in a local infection and adenopathy presumably caused by a virus. Although the use of tetracycline has been advocated for this infection, Carithers et al.[19] state that no antibiotic has much value, and that it is usually a mild, self-limited problem.

VENOMOUS SNAKE BITES

Agreement on the treatment of these injuries is less than universal. Snyder,[20] on the basis of a large personal experience, has outlined six useful steps:

1. Try to get a positive identification of the snake.
2. Outline the bites as clearly as possible. The extremity may be cooled but freezing should be assiduously avoided.

3. If a large snake caused extensive trauma and severe envenomation, give Antivenin (Crotalidae) Polyvalent (Wyeth) diluted with 100 ml. of normal saline containing 100 mg. of hydrocortisone (Solu-Cortef) intra-arterially over a 20-minute period. The amount of Antivenin administered should be two to nine vials depending on the severity of the envenomation. Inject into a large artery just proximal to the bite (e.g., the brachial artery in wounds of the hand); a tourniquet should be loosely applied above the injection site before injection. Antivenin is provoked in horses and appropriate precautions should be taken for hypersensitivity reactions to horse serum.
4. The bite wound should be incised or, if quite severe, excised and the venom "milked" out. The wound is left open, of course. Be careful not to injure underlying structures when incising or excising.
5. Give ancillary support.
6. Hospitalize the patient.

SPIDER AND SCORPION BITES

These injuries may or may not cause significant local injury. Black widow spider and scorpion bites result mainly in systemic problems. These bites are treated locally with cold compresses, immobilization, and analgesics. The systemic effects may be great and are well-outlined in the *Handbook of Poisoning*.[21]

The brown or recluse spider inflicts a bite that may cause significant local necrosis requiring eventual wide excision and skin grafting. Therefore, patients with recluse spider bites should be watched for a skin slough at the bite site. This spider bite may also cause hemolysis systemically. As always, the injured part should be immobilized and elevated. Close observation, sometimes with hospitalization, is indicated.

REFERENCES

1. Bell, M. S.: The changing pattern of pyogenic infections of the hand. Hand, 8:298–302, 1976.

2. Eaton, R. G., and Butsch, D. P.: Antibiotic guidelines for hand infections. Surg. Gynecol. Obstet., *130*:119–122, 1970.

3. Stone, N. H., et al.: Empirical selection of antibiotics for hand infections. J. Bone Joint Surg., *51A*:899–903, 1969.

4. Wilkowske, C. J., and Hermans, P. E.: Actions and uses of antimicrobial agents in the treatment of musculoskeletal infections. Orthop. Clin. North Am., 6:1129–1144, 1975.

5. Barlow, A. J. E., et al.: Chronic paronychia. Br. J. Dermatol., *82*:448–453, 1970.

6. Linscheid, R. L., and Dobyns, J. H.: Common and uncommon infections of the hand. Orthop. Clin. North Am., 6:1063–1104, 1975.

7. Kilgore, E. S., et al.: Treatment of felons. Am. J. Surg., *130*:194–198, 1975.

8. Lampe, E. W.: Surgical Anatomy of the Hand. CIBA Symposium, CIBA Pharmaceutical Co., Summit, New Jersey, 1969.

9. Kelly, P. J.: Bacterial arthritis in the adult. Orthop. Clin. North Am., 6:973–981, 1975.

10. Sim, F. H.: Anaerobic infections. Orthop. Clin. North Am., 6:1049–1056, 1975.

11. Anderson, C. B., et al.: Anaerobic streptococcal infections simulating gas gangrene. Arch. Surg., *104*:186–189, 1972.

12. Van Beek, A., et al.: Nonclostridial gas forming infections. Arch. Surg., *108*:552–557, 1974.

13. Giuliano, A., et al.: Bacteriology of necrotizing fasciitis. Am. J. Surg., *134*:52–57, 1977.

14. Baxter, C. R.: Surgical management of soft tissue infections. Surg. Clin. North Am., 52:1483–1499, 1972.

15. Oill, P. A., et al.: Infectious disease emergencies. Part V. Patients presenting with localized infections. West. J. Med., *126*:196–208, 1977.

16. Williams, C. S., and Riordan, D. C.: Mycobacterium marinum (atypical acid-fast bacillus) infections of the hand. J. Bone Joint Surg., 55A:1042–1050, 1973.

17. Duran, R. J., et al.: Sporotrichosis. A report of twenty-three cases in the upper extremity. J. Bone Joint Surg., 39A:1330–1342, 1957.

18. Mann, R. J., et al.: Human bites of the hand: Twenty years' experience. J. Hand Surg., 2:97–104, 1977.

19. Carithers, H. A., et al.: Cat scratch disease. Its natural history. JAMA, 207:312–316, 1969.

20. Snyder, C. C., et al.: The snakebitten hand. Plast. Reconstr. Surg., 49:275–281, 1972.

21. Dreisbach, R. H.: Handbook of Poisoning. 9th ed. Los Altos, Calif., Lange Medical Publications, 1977. pp. 454–462.

9

Tendon Injuries

T ENDONS are glistening white, relatively inert structures that provide a source of endless fascination for students of the hand. Perhaps no biologic system appears quite so elegant and beautiful when one has the unusual opportunity to observe it function in vivo. Tendons are the agents of muscular activity—the direct movers of the joints. If a tendon should become disrupted, stuck, or lose its angle of pull for any cause whatsoever, it will function poorly or not at all, and the muscle that motivates the tendon will have no function to perform. The joints ordinarily moved by the nonfunctional tendon will cease to act in at least one direction, and may even become stiff.

Mechanisms of Injury

Tendon function is lost most frequently by disruption, usually as a result of trauma, although rupture from disease is not uncommon. Lacerations are the most common cause of traumatic disruption, but tendons may be torn or avulsed as well. Tendon malfunction due to loss of gliding ability may be caused by scar formation from injuries to adjacent structures as well as from injuries to the tendon itself. Healing fractures often cause this type of malfunction. Tendons may become stuck in their natural tunnels or sheaths owing to a variety of causes.

Tendons may lose their mechanical advantage because of loss of pulleys, so that all their motion is then expended on "bowstringing" rather than on moving joints. In normal hands, tendons pass through fibro-osseous tunnels at or near certain joints.

135

These tunnels serve functionally as pulleys and prevent the tendon from bowstringing. This concept can be better understood if you imagine a simple hinge joint that is arranged to move from full extension of 180 degrees to flexion of 90 degrees. If a tendon crosses this joint without any restraint as it contracts and flexes the joint, it will bend to form the third side of a triangle. Biologically this is not an efficient design because a very loose skin envelope would be required to accommodate this tendon as it arches between the two bones (or becomes a "bowstring" across them). This arrangement would also require a huge tendon excursion to achieve maximal flexion. However, if the tendon is restrained near the joint by a tunnel that still allows almost frictionless sliding, bowstringing across the joint will not occur and the excursion required of the tendon is much less. This latter system is the normal one.

The tendon problem encountered most frequently, especially in an emergency setting, is disruption from laceration; most of this chapter is devoted to this topic. However, a primary care physician may be called upon to diagnose tendon malfunction due to loss of glide in natural sheaths and disruption due to closed trauma or disease; these conditions are also discussed.

Pathologic conditions may affect the 24 extrinsic tendons of the hand anywhere along their course. In general, problems affecting intrinsic musculotendinous units usually arise within the muscles, although injury to isolated intrinsic tendons may occur. In the digits, extrinsic and intrinsic tendons combine dorsally to form the extensor mechanism, which is frequently injured.

Accurate, early diagnosis of problems affecting the tendons is important. In many cases, a delay in diagnosis, treatment, or referral to a hand specialist may jeopardize the chances for maximal recovery of function.

OPEN TENDON INJURIES

These are the injuries seen most often in the office and emergency department. The injury may be large or small, tidy or untidy, or associated with skin loss or injury to deep structures. When a laceration or wound overlies a tendon, the probability that the tendon has been injured is great, and the burden of disproving the presence of tendon injury lies with the examining physician. This is especially important when the injury involves the dorsum of the hand, because the tendons are so superficial in this location. Accurate determination of the mechanism of injury is important in assessing the likelihood of tendon injury.

CLOSED TENDON INJURIES

These injuries are less common but more subtle than open tendon injuries. The violence done to a part may be minimal or maximal. Often patients cannot articulate the nature of the problem—they just know that some part "is not working right." Ruptures of tendons may occur during normal activity in patients whose tendons have been weakened by disease (e.g., rheumatoid arthritis) or previous injury.

Diagnosis of Tendon Injuries

Tendon injuries are diagnosed by the same sequential steps that have been discussed in Chapter 2. Observation of the quiescent hand often suffices to make the diagnosis (Fig. 9-1). Testing for active function is important in tendon injuries; a review of the functional anatomy of tendons (Chapter 1) may be in order.

Testing for sensibility, although giving no direct information about tendon injury, is important because digital nerves are often injured when flexor tendons have been lacerated. Finally, direct examination is important, especially with extensor tendons, because the juncturae tendinum (Fig. 9-2) may allow weak digital extension even if the tendon has been lacerated. Direct examination on the flexor side sometimes reveals partially lacerated tendons that might rupture if not repaired.

Treatment of Tendon Injuries

To some extent this depends on the experience and inclination of the primary care physician and on the availability of expert

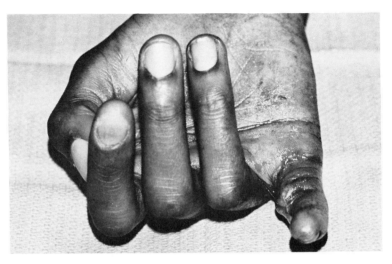

FIG. 9-1. *The diagnosis of this young woman's problem may be made by observation alone: both flexor tendons are lacerated.*

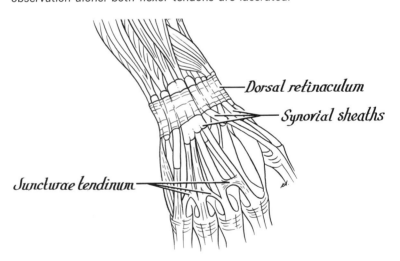

Dorsal retinaculum

Synovial sheaths

Juncturae tendinum

The extrinsic extensor tendons

FIG. 9-2. *The juncturae tendinum should be noted and their importance understood.*

help. Certainly in large metropolitan centers where hand specialists are readily available for consultation, most patients with tendon injuries should be referred to these specialists. However, when injured tendons are easily accessible and reparable in minimal time, they may be treated in the office or emergency room. In practical terms, such conditions occur only with some extensor tendon injuries. When tendon injuries cannot be repaired immediately, consultation with a hand surgeon should be sought, the skin should be sutured, and the hand supported with a forearm splint. Although it may be appropriate to delay referral to a hand specialist for one or two days, consultation with a hand surgeon should take place at the time of the initial examination of the patient.

Specific Tendon Injuries

It is most convenient and useful to discuss both flexor and extensor tendon injuries by anatomic location. In each case, four questions will be considered:

1. What is the normal and pathologic anatomy?
2. Is the pathologic change a consequence of an open injury, a closed injury, or a disease process?
3. How can one diagnose the injury most expeditiously?
4. How should one handle the injury in the emergency setting?

EXTENSOR TENDON INJURIES

At the level of the dorsal forearm, wrist, and hand, extensor tendons are discrete and obvious. At the level of the MCP joint, it is proper to speak of the dorsal tendinous structure as the extensor mechanism. The extensor mechanism is a broad, flat aponeurotic band composed of extrinsic extensor tendon and the lateral bands formed by the tendons of the lumbrical and interossei muscles; in the little finger and thumb the border intrinsic tendons are also included in the extensor mechanism. It is important to understand that the intrinsic tendons are the primary extensors of the IP joints of digits II through V, while the extrinsic tendons exert their primary force at the MCP joints. The intrinsic tendons lie volar to the axis of motion of the MCP joints and are actually MCP flexors. They lie dorsal to the axis of motion of the PIP and DIP joints and are, therefore, extensors of those joints. If the tendons shift in regard to these axes, a pathologic situation exists.

In the thumb the same general anatomic situation exists, but with an important exception. The thumb has an extrinsic extensor that exerts its force on the distal phalanx; namely, the extensor pollicis longus. Loss of this tendon will prevent forcible extension, and hyperextension at the IP joint in particular. The IP joint can still be extended weakly by virtue of the intrinsic tendons. (You are encouraged to review the functional anatomy of the extensor mechanism in Chapter 1 to firmly understand the following.)

It is far easier to analyze extensor injuries if one considers the following six extensor zones (Fig. 9-3): I, the dorsal finger at the DIP joint; II, the dorsal finger at the PIP joint and the thumb at the IP joint; III, dorsal digit except at joints; IV, the dorsal hand; V, the dorsal wrist; VI, the dorsal forearm.

EXTENSOR ZONE I

Injury to the extensor mechanism here causes a deformity known as a *baseball* or *mallet finger* (Fig. 9-4). The tendon inserts into the distal phalanx at the proximal dorsal lip. It may be avulsed from the bone, lacerated near the insertion, or come off with a piece of bone. The most common cause of a mallet finger is a closed, often apparently trivial injury. Somewhat more forceful trauma may cause a dorsal lip fracture. Less common is mallet deformity due to a laceration, and rupture of the tendon at this joint because of arthritis is uncommon.

Diagnosis is made by observing the obviously drooping distal phalanx and noting that it cannot be actively extended. If trauma of any violence is suspected, a roentgenogram should be taken. If there is laceration, inspect the tendon directly.

Management of mallet deformity due to a fracture is outlined in Chapter 10. A closed mallet deformity should be treated by application of a splint to hold the DIP in full extension (Fig. 9-5A)

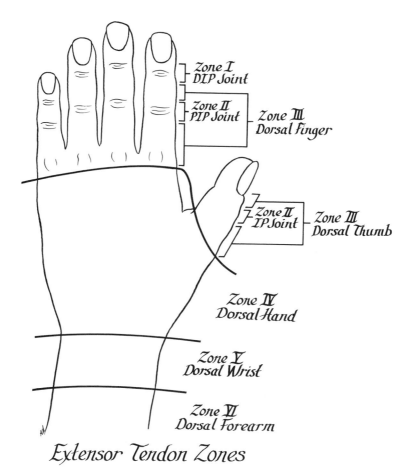

Zone I
DIP Joint

Zone II
PIP Joint

Zone III
Dorsal Finger

Zone II
IP Joint

Zone III
Dorsal Thumb

Zone IV
Dorsal Hand

Zone V
Dorsal Wrist

Zone VI
Dorsal Forearm

Extensor Tendon Zones

FIG. 9-3. *It is useful to place extensor tendon injuries in one of these zones for treatment and prognosis.*

and yet allow free PIP motion (Fig. 9-5B). The joint should be supported in full extension *at all times* for eight weeks. The patient can learn to change his own splint, but during changes he must either hold the joint up with the other hand or support it on a firm surface, The splint may be shifted from the dorsal to the volar surface to avoid skin maceration, but the dorsal position is most satisfactory and should be used most of the time.

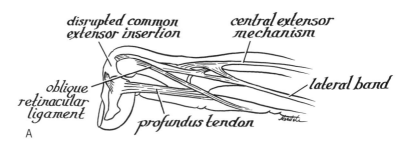

disrupted common
extensor insertion

central extensor
mechanism

oblique
retinacular
ligament

lateral band

profundus tendon

A

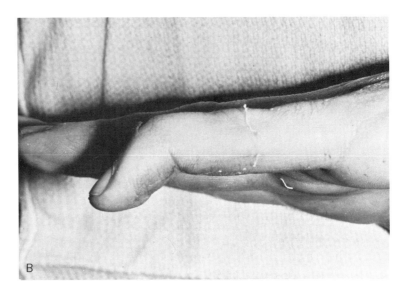

B

FIG. 9-4.   (A) The mallet finger injury. (B) This mallet deformity was caused by a laceration, but the appearance in profile is the same as with a closed mallet injury.

With mallet deformity caused by open injury, the joint should be fixed in full extension with an 0.035-inch Kirschner wire, Concept wire, or the equivalent. The tendon is then sutured with 5-0 nylon. Use of clear nylon may be advisable because black, blue, or green sutures may be visible through the thin skin. The pin is left in place for six to eight weeks.

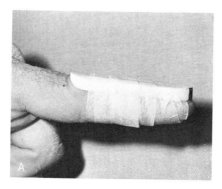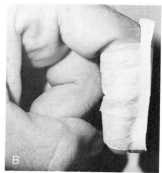

FIG. 9-5.   *(A) The mallet splint. (B) The mallet splint should allow free PIP flexion.*

EXTENSOR ZONE II

Any injury to the extensor mechanism at this level may allow the lateral bands to slip volar to the axis of joint motion and paradoxically become flexors of the PIP joint instead of extensors (Figs. 9-6 and 9-7). This is known as the *boutonniere* or *buttonhole* deformity of the PIP joint.

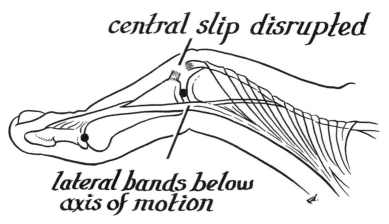

central slip disrupted

lateral bands below axis of motion

FIG. 9-6.   *In closed injuries, boutonniere deformity is probably potential rather than actual due to attenuation of the extensor mechanism over the PIP joint.*

The cause of a boutonniere deformity may be a laceration, but more commonly it is a direct blow over the dorsal joint or indirect violence to the finger with consequent injury to the extensor mechanism. This defect may also occur with longstanding rheumatoid arthritis.

Diagnosis is made by observing the typical stance of the digit (see Fig. 9-7). In an acute closed injury, swelling about the PIP joint may be so great that a definite diagnosis is difficult. In this situation, the often-present hyperextension stance of the DIP joint may provide a clue to the diagnosis. Usually, however, the examiner will have to exercise a high degree of suspicion and assume that the patient has either an actual or potential boutonniere deformity and treat accordingly.

Management of an acute closed boutonniere deformity, actual or potential, involves the application of a splint that holds the PIP joint in full extension while leaving the MCP and DIP joints free to move (Fig. 9-8). If the deformity is caused by laceration of the extensor mechanism, suture the tendons with running 5-0 nylon and apply a PIP extension splint. Volar application of the splint for the first few days may be more practical when a wound is present.

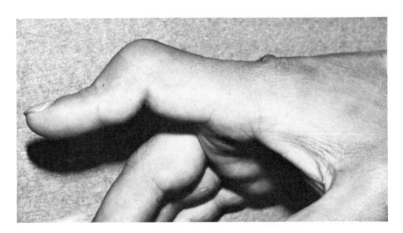

FIG. 9-7. This young man has an established boutonniere deformity. Note the hyperextended DIP joint. This probably could have been prevented by early correct splinting.

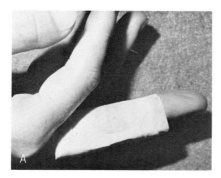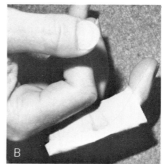

FIG. 9-8. *(A) The boutonniere splint, with PIP joint extension. (B) The boutonniere splint should allow flexion of MCP and DIP joints.*

Boutonniere deformities treated in this fashion for about four weeks usually resolve satisfactorily. If neglected, the deformity may become fixed, and secondary reconstruction is complicated and often not successful. The joint need not be supported with quite the same consistency required for a mallet deformity, but the splint should be worn most of the day and always at night. It may be removed only for bathing and washing. Any patient with a boutonniere deformity should be referred to a hand surgeon for follow-up if feasible.

EXTENSOR ZONE III

This zone includes the extensor mechanism from the point where it broadens out at the MCP joints and over the digits except at IP joints. It is a broad, flat band that hugs the digital bones dorsally. Injury is usually due to laceration; partial laceration is common (Fig. 9-9). Diagnosis is made by direct inspection. Treatment involves repair with a running 5-0 nylon suture, and placing the injured finger and an adjacent digit in a short arm cast or splint for about 10 to 14 days with wrist extended, MCPs flexed and IPs nearly straight. Thereafter the patient should use a finger guard of the four-prong variety (see Chapter 4) for another 10 days while working and sleeping.

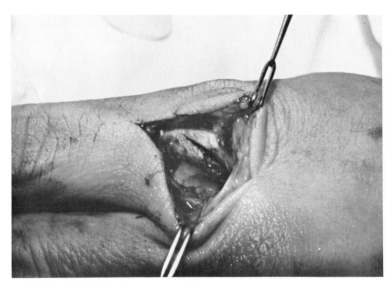

FIG. 9-9. *This Zone III laceration injury is common and can be diagnosed only by direct examination.*

EXTENSOR ZONE IV

Eight tendons traverse the dorsal hand from wrist to digits. Those to digits II through V are connected by bands called juncturae tendinum (see Fig. 9-2). As in the digits, the tendons here are superficial, covered only with thin fascia and loose areolar tissue. The closer to the wrist that a laceration occurs, the more likely is the proximal stump to retract because tendon amplitude increases proximally. As shown in Figure 9-10, retraction of a proximal stump may present a substantial problem.

Injuries at this level are usually caused by open injury, commonly lacerations. Diagnosis can be made by functional tests and direct examination. No matter what results are obtained from functional tests, always suspect tendon laceration when treating dorsal wounds until you can see the intact tendon.

If the two tendon ends can be readily retrieved, repair may be carried out with a 4-0 nylon suture utilizing either of the tech-

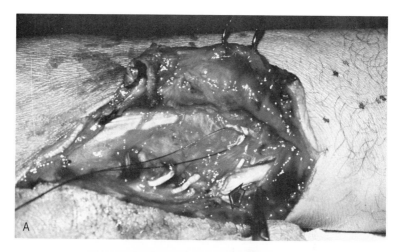

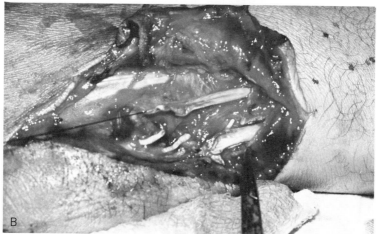

FIG. 9-10.   (A) *This photograph shows a dorsal hand laceration. The fingers are to the left of the photograph. The arrow points to the extensor carpi ulnaris, which has been sutured. At the top of the wound is the extensor digitorum communis slip to the ring finger. The two divided tendons in the middle of the distal wound are the communis and proprius tendons to the little finger; the proximal, retracted ends of these tendons are attached to the suture. (B) The retracted tendon ends have been pulled down.*

niques shown in Figure 9-11. In areas where expert help is available, it may be the wiser course to refer these patients to specialists, but certainly repair in emergency department or office is
often feasible. The case illustrated in Figure 9-10 was repaired in
the operating room. The more proximal the tendon laceration
occurs, the more likely is the necessity for repair under regional or
general anesthesia.

Following repair, a cast or splint is applied with the wrist in
extension and with MCP and IP joints slightly flexed (about 20 to
25 degrees). The IP joints may be left free dorsally but supported
volarly to prevent forced flexion. If a tendon to digits II through V
is lacerated, all digits should be included in the cast or splint. If a
thumb tendon is lacerated, only the thumb need be included in
the cast or splint.

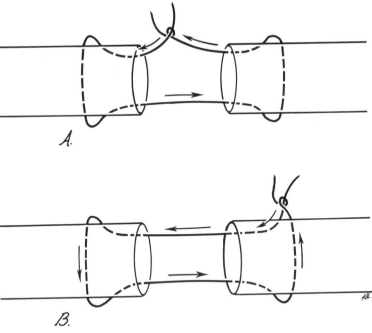

A.

B.

FIG. 9-11. *Either of these techniques of tendon suture serve well to repair extensor tendons in Zone IV.*

EXTENSOR ZONES V AND VI

The wrist (Zone V) is the only area in which the extensor tendons lie in synovial lined compartments, of which there are six. The amplitude of the tendons at this level is large, and retraction of the stumps usually occurs in case of separation. The low forearm (Zone VI) is free of synovial compartments, but the tendons here lie fairly deep and are difficult to expose.

Injury at these levels may be due to laceration or rupture from disease or old trauma. Laceration is probably the most common cause of injury, but rupture from rheumatoid synovitis is fairly common. Rupture—especially of the extensor pollicis longus— may follow a Colles' fracture.

In almost all instances, patients with tendon injuries in these zones should be referred to a hand surgeon for repair.

FLEXOR TENDON INJURIES

The flexor tendons of the hand and their repair after injury have been the subjects of much lively debate among hand surgeons for many years. The flexor system is less subtle than the extensor system. The tendons are round or elliptical structures from beginning to end. They do not combine with intrinsics to form complicated mechanisms in the digits. When digital flexors are divided, the entire interphalangeal flexion mechanism fails and the lack is painfully apparent (see Fig. 9-1). The flexors, in comparison with the extensors, are deep structures that have a large amplitude of glide in the digit, so they frequently retract a long distance when lacerated. These tendons are closely associated with nerves throughout their entire length, and combined injury of both structures is common. For much of their length the flexors lie in synovial lined sheaths; infections, especially in the digital sheath, are common and serious.

The flexor tendons are most easily considered when they are placed in five different zones (Fig. 9-12): I, the distal one and one-half phalanges; II, the midpalm to the middle of the middle phalanx (this is the notorious "No Man's Land") III, the distal end of the carpal tunnel to the midpalm; IV, the carpal tunnel; V, the wrist and low forearm.

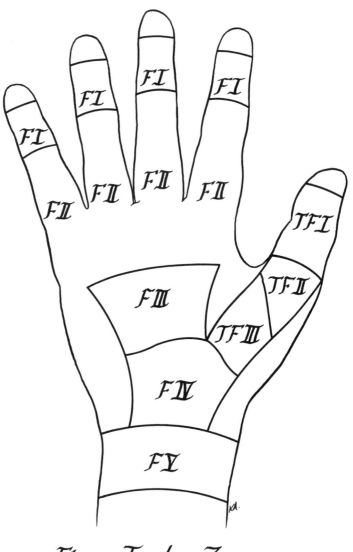

Flexor Tendon Zones

FIG. 9-12. As with the extensors, it is useful to place flexor tendon injuries in one of these zones.

FLEXOR ZONE I

The profundus tendon is alone in this area; the sublimis tendon inserts at the distal end of Zone II. The digital thecal sheath ends approximately at the DIP joint. The profundus tendon inserts into the proximal volar portion of the distal phalanx. A short, thick band just proximal to its insertion is called the short vinculum; this is a mesentery through which the tendon receives a significant part of its blood supply.

Problems in this area are most often due to open injuries; knife and glass lacerations are especially common. Closed traumatic ruptures of the tendon may occur following intense local pressure on a flexed distal phalanx (Fig. 9-13). This injury occurs most commonly, but by no means exclusively, in young men. Rupture of the tendon due to disease is uncommon.

Diagnosis is made primarily by functional examination. Direct examination may be necessary to diagnose a partial tendon laceration. A patient with an obvious tendon laceration or rupture should be referred to a hand surgeon. It is best to arrange a

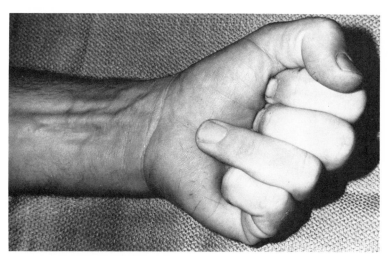

FIG. 9-13. *This young man ruptured his flexor digitorum profundus of his ring finger at its insertion while scuffling with some assailants.*

consultation as soon as possible, although repair may be delayed up to one or two weeks without jeopardizing the chances for a successful repair. If repair is to be delayed, it is best to close the skin, apply a good dressing and splint, and take other appropriate steps to minimize the chances of swelling and infection.

If the tendon is partially lacerated and the laceration can be exposed easily, repair with a mattress suture of 4-0 nylon should be done. The hand and one or more digits are then put in a cast with the wrist and MCP joints in flexion and the IP joints in slight flexion. Remember that the three ulnar profundi tendons have a common muscle belly, and these tendons should always be treated as a unit. If a partial laceration cannot be visualized easily, the patient should be treated as though a complete division exists. Partial lacerations may presage complete rupture, especially if unguarded digital use is permitted.

FLEXOR ZONE II

This is the most common area of injury to flexor tendons. Its descriptive term "No Man's Land" has been attributed to the pioneer hand surgeon, Sterling Bunnell, the implication being that no man (i.e., surgeon) should venture into this area unprepared for the difficulties to be encountered. The belief that repair of flexor tendons in this zone should never be a primary procedure has changed considerably in the past 20 years, and primary or delayed primary repairs are now done routinely.

A brief review of Chapter 1 will remind you that two tendons, each with a large amplitude or glide, are snugly contained in a synovial sheath in this zone. At the proximal end of the sheath, the sublimis tendon lies superficial to the profundus tendon. Midway in the sheath the sublimis tendon decussates, and each of the decussating slips wraps around the profundus and inserts at the proximal volar portion of the middle phalanx. The insertion is actually both long and broad and commences at the distal end of the proximal phalanx. The sublimis tendon also has a short vinculum, and several long vinculae perforate the sublimis from the area of its short vinculum to provide an additional blood supply to the profundus tendon.

Any injury or disease that interferes with these finely tuned mechanisms may cause problems with digital flexion. Perforating small objects may lead to infection (see Chapter 8). Diseases such as rheumatoid arthritis may cause tendon constriction and eventual rupture of the tendons. The most common cause of problems in this area is laceration, following which retraction of one or both tendons occurs frequently. Partially lacerated tendons may interfere with their normal gliding.

Diagnosis of tendon injuries in this area may often be made by simple observation (see Fig. 9-1). Functional examination may be helpful, and occasionally direct examination is necessary. Sensibility should always be tested because digital nerves are frequently injured along with these tendons.

Any injury and most diseases afflicting tendons in this area should be promptly referred to a hand surgeon. Once a diagnosis of partial or total laceration in flexor Zone II has been made, repair moves beyond the scope of the emergency department or office. As with Zone I injuries, repair may be delayed for a few days.

FLEXOR ZONE III

This is a rather small zone but it contains many critically important structures. It comprises the area between the distal end of the carpal tunnel and the entrance to the flexor tendon sheaths. The tendons are free of synovial sheath in this zone. At the proximal end of the zone the superficial transverse arterial arch crosses the tendons, giving off the common digital arteries. Between the arterial arch and the tendons, the median nerve separates into its terminal sensory branches.

Tendon damage in this zone is almost always due to penetrating trauma. Isolated tendon damage is unlikely in this zone; significant nerve and vascular injury usually occur concurrently. When porcelain faucet handles were in common use injury in this zone was seen more frequently, caused by penetration of porcelain pieces following a forceful blow to an unyielding handle.

For practical purposes, diagnosis of injuries in this zone is made by observation and functional examination. A careful sensory examination should always be done. Although direct examination may be helpful occasionally, it may just compound the problem with potential wound contamination without materially aiding the diagnosis.

Management in the primary care setting is by suturing the skin and immediate referral to a hand surgeon. If at all possible, this type of injury should be surgically repaired within the first few hours after injury.

FLEXOR ZONE IV

This is the carpal tunnel zone, which runs from the wrist crease to the cardinal or thumb line (see Chapter 1). Nine flexor tendons lie deep to the median nerve in this synovium-lined tunnel.

Tendon abnormalities in this zone are uncommon. Injury may occur from penetrating trauma, but this is unusual because of the thick volar protection provided by the volar carpal ligament, the palmar fascia, and the thick palmar skin. Tendon rupture due to synovial proliferative disease may be seen occasionally.

Diagnosis is made by observation of the quiescent hand and functional examination. Because of the close proximity of the median nerve, a thorough sensory evaluation should be made. Management is by referral to a specialist.

FLEXOR ZONE V

This zone runs from the musculotendinous junctions to the carpal tunnel entrance. The tendons and the median nerve are quite superficial in this area, being covered only by thin volar skin and thin antebrachial fascia. Some synovium encloses the tendons in this zone. With injury, the synovium becomes edematous, making identification of tendons difficult.

Open injuries are by far the most common cause of tendon problems in this area. The injury may be caused by any sharp object, but one should be especially wary of injuries caused by glass, because the shards can spare surface structures while penetrating and wreaking havoc on deeper structures. Always assume the worst with glass lacerations.

Diagnosis is made by the four modalities of examination (observation, functional evaluation, sensibility testing, and direct examination). Since median and ulnar nerve injuries often (indeed usually) accompany wrist lacerations, the sensory examination is important. If the palmaris longus tendon is intact on direct examination, you have some justification for assuming that no deep injury has occurred. If it is lacerated, you should assume that deep structures have been injured, even if the examination is equivocal or otherwise indicates no injury. (See Figs. 14-2 and 14-3B.)

Any injury in this zone should be explored operatively, and early referral to a specialist is in order. A delay of several days in surgical repair is not serious if careful wound toilet and proper dressing techniques are performed.

THE THUMB

The flexor zones of the thumb apply fairly closely but not exactly with those of the other digits. Zone I is the same as for the other digits. Zone II contains only the flexor pollicis longus, but otherwise no significant difference exists. Zone III is somewhat different, because the flexor pollicis longus tendon lies beneath the thenar musculature in this area rather than relatively free, as occurs in the palm. Zones IV and V follow the same pattern as the tendons of the other four digits.

Tendon Constriction Syndromes

Wherever a tendon passes through a tendon sheath, the potential exists for constriction and binding of the tendon, preventing glide. In actual practice, this condition occurs often enough in certain areas to merit an eponym. Medically the disorder is known as a stenosing tenosynovitis.

The most common stenosing tenosynovitis affects the digital flexors in the proximal portion of Zone II. The patient is said to have a trigger finger (or trigger thumb). The digit usually goes into flexion easily enough but extends with a painful, almost audible snap. Pain is often referred to the dorsal PIP joint (or IP in the thumb), although the problem exists in the volar palm. It occurs most often in the early morning, after the digits have been quiet for several hours. The finger may actually become "locked" in flexion.

Injection of about 0.5 to 1.0 ml. of a cortisone-lidocaine combination into the tendon sheath will usually "unlock" the tendon and relieve pain. The best technique is to insert a no. 27 half-inch (12.5-mm.) needle into the palm at the level of the proximal tendon sheath to the depth of the bone (gently!!). Then withdraw the syringe, keeping a steady pressure on the plunger. As the needle tip enters the free tendon sheath, the fluid squirts out. The patient will have a sensation of the finger "filling up." Interestingly, the "click" is usually accentuated after the injection and the patient should be warned of this. The patient should also be advised that further injections or even surgical release may be necessary, and follow-up arrangements should be made. The IP joints should be splinted in extension for about one week following the injection.

The first dorsal compartment, through which pass the extensor pollicis brevis and slips of the abductor pollicis longus, is prone to a stenotic condition known as DeQuervain's stenosing tenosynovitis (Fig. 9-14A). The simplest test for this is the Finkelstein test:

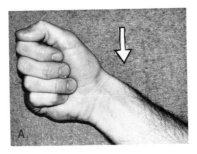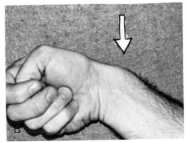

FIG. 9-14.   (A) *The arrow points to the first dorsal compartment, where the extensor pollicis brevis and abductor pollicis longus become constricted in DeQuervain's stenosing tenosynovitis. (B) In the Finkelstein test for diagnosis of DeQuervain's disease, pain occurs in the first compartment when the thumb is grasped and the wrist deviated ulnarly.*

the thumb is grasped by the other four digits and the wrist deviated ulnarly (Fig. 9-14B). Pain in the first dorsal compartment with this maneuver constitutes a positive result. Injection with 2 ml. of a cortisone-lidocaine mixture, using a no. 25, one-inch needle, into the compartment and splinting the wrist and thumb for one week are recommended. Whenever cortisone is injected into the dorsal hand or wrist, the patient, especially those with dark skins, should be warned that depigmentation may occur.

One other rather curious disorder exists that has at least an anatomic association with DeQuervain's tenosynovitis. This is crepitation of the muscle bellies of the extensor pollicis brevis and the abductor pollicis longus; it is called myositis crepitans. The patient complains of pain and tenderness and the examiner feels a crepitation of the muscle bellies when the tendons are actively moved. Administration of an oral anti-inflammatory drug such as phenylbutazone and immobilization for a few days are usually curative.

Other tendon stenoses are encountered less frequently. In any area, discrete injections of cortisone, immobilization, and administration of an oral anti-inflammatory drug will relieve pain pending more definitive treatment if that proves necessary.

REFERENCES

1. Conolly, W. B., and Kilgore, E. S., Jr.: Tendons. pp. 162–211. *In* The Hand: Surgical and Non-Surgical Management. Kilgore, E. S., Jr., and Graham, W. P., III (eds.), Philadelphia, Lea & Febiger, 1977.

2. AAOS Symposium on Tendon Surgery in the Hand. St. Louis, C. V. Mosby, 1975.

10

Bone and Joint Injuries

njuries to the hand's skeletal framework are common, accounting for about 10% of all hand injuries.[1] These injuries include those to bones, to the joints at which they articulate, and to the ligaments that hold the bones together. Skeletal injuries usually involve some injury to the surrounding soft tissues. Often this involves a compromise of vascular perfusion because of swelling, which will resolve with proper treatment of the skeletal lesion. In some skeletal injuries, especially those that are open, major independent structures may be significantly stretched or disrupted, and one may find accompanying nerve, tendon, or skin injury. As has been emphasized previously, it is important to treat the entire hand and not just isolated tissue systems. Our goal is always to achieve maximal function in minimal time with a minimal number of procedures.

Bone Injury

The usual significant injury to a bone is fracture. Clinical diagnosis is often easy on the basis of the history and physical examination, but a roentgenogram is essential to confirm the diagnosis and analyze the extent of injury.

When considering bone injury in the hand, it is useful to consider the bones in three categories (Fig. 10-1): the long bones, the carpals, and the distal phalanges. The long bones (which include the two forearm bones, radius and ulna, all the metacarpals, all the proximal phalanges and all the middle phalanges), are strut bones that elongate the digits so they may, in conjunction with the

158

joints, both extend and flex as well as perform adduction and abduction. To perform adequately the bones must be able to extend and flex in a coordinated fashion. If there is a significant rotary or bowing deformity, the involved digit will either be unable to flex and extend in its normal arc or will do so in a crooked and uncoordinated fashion (Fig. 10-2). Therefore, with fractures of these bones the goal must be to prevent rotary or bowing deformities that will interfere with function. This demands good alignment and good stability. Alignment is necessary for healing in the proper position, and stability is necessary so that the period of immobilization will not have to be overly extended.

Some fractures are inherently better aligned and more stable than others. In general, comminuted and open fractures are less likely to be stable than simple and closed fractures. A midshaft

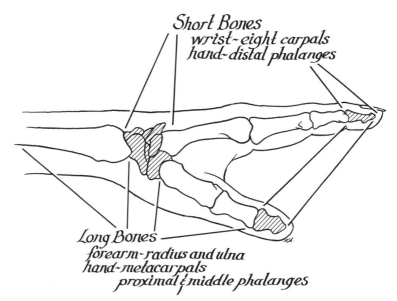

Short Bones
wrist-eight carpals
hand-distal phalanges

Long Bones
forearm-radius and ulna
hand-metacarpals
proximal & middle phalanges

FIG. 10-1. *This is a useful way to think of the bones. The long bones are all strut bones that elongate the forearm, hand, or digits, thereby providing the length element necessary for function. The wrist bones allow great arcs of motion, yet they can be firmly stabilized. The distal phalanges provide firm supports for the sensitive fingerpads.*

fracture will probably present less of a problem than one that is intra-articular. Many long-bone fractures of the hand can be treated by reduction and fixation with a cast or splint. However, hand surgeons tend increasingly to fix fractures of these bones internally, so that early mobilization can be started, and final mobility is much better than that attained with closed treatment.

The second category of bones is the carpals. These eight little bones (or really seven bones if one considers the pisiform as a type of sesamoid) connect the long forearm bones to the metacarpals forming the "wrist" joint. The unique feature of the carpus is that it permits a remarkable range of motion of the hand on the forearm, yet it can be fixed and rigidly held to provide great strength. Isolated injuries to the carpal bones usually result in long-term problems because of pain due to nonhealing and loss of mobility due to interference with joint function (i.e., loss of smooth, full glide between bones). The carpus must be considered as a unit that comprises both bones and joints because it is difficult to separate the two structures.

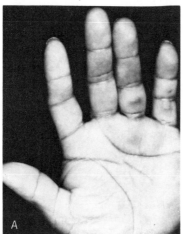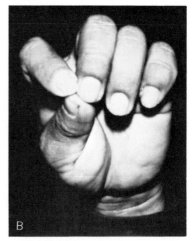

FIG. 10-2. (A) This middle-aged man has a healed fracture of his second metacarpal. The hand looks normal with digital extension. However, with digital flexion (B), the same hand has an obvious deformity of the index ray. Although this was not disabling, a similar deformity in a central ray might have been.

The third category of bones includes the distal phalanges. These little bones need to provide pain-free support for the highly sensible fingerpads. Pain-free union usually occurs if there is no infection. Special situations involving these bones are discussed under specific injuries.

Joint Injuries

A joint is the junction between two or more bones and the associated tissues that permit or prevent motion of those bones. Supporting structures include true ligaments, fibrous plates (which are really thickened ligaments), and tendon insertions. The joint may also have a thin, fibrous capsule, which offers little actual support. Articulating bones are covered with articular cartilage, and the recesses of the joint are lined with synovium, which provides lubrication for the joint.

A joint is disabled because it becomes immobile, too mobile, dislocated, or painful. Joints may be injured by infection (see Chapter 8), by disease (see Chapter 15), or most commonly by trauma. Injury may be due to indirect violence of twisting, wrenching, compression, or distraction. Joints may also be injured by direct penetrating trauma that directly injures one or more of the various components of the joint. The result may range from a traumatic synovitis to total joint destruction. The supporting structures or ligaments are composed of firm, white tissue of varying thickness and limited elasticity. When torn, they may become interposed between bone ends, making closed reduction impossible. When they are stretched or torn, the body will respond by producing a protein-rich exudate that subsides only to leave a permanent residue of stiffness.

Principles of Treating Bone and Joint Injuries

For the primary care physician, the most basic principle is to diagnose the injury accurately. Many bone and joint injuries are easily overlooked or misdiagnosed.[2] A careful history should be taken to elicit any account of twisting or wrenching trauma. The injured part should be examined carefully. Is the joint just a bit crooked? Why doesn't it rotate fully? Why is the wrist so painful? The answers to these and any other pertinent questions should be sought.

The roentgenogram is the essential diagnostic tool in bone and joint injuries. Proper views should be obtained (see specific injuries). Be especially mindful of not allowing the technician to overlap fingers on a lateral view (Fig. 10-3). The physician should always examine the roentgenogram and not accept just a report. If there is any doubt about injury to a structure, obtain more views and get comparison studies of the opposite, uninjured extremity or part of the extremity.

If a firm diagnosis can be made, and if the fracture or dislocation can be reduced easily and is stable after reduction, you have rendered definitive treatment. Reduction should be done under anesthesia, which in the office or emergency department comprises limited regional block or, occasionally, direct infiltration of lidocaine. An appropriate cast or splint is then applied.

If a firm diagnosis can be made but the injury is unstable and/or irreducible, the injured part should be immobilized with a

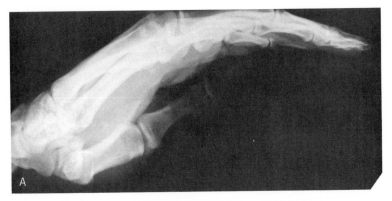

FIG. 10-3. *(A) Unless you specify "isolated lateral views of the digits" on the roentgenogram request, you will have trouble deciphering the superimposed images on the developed picture.*

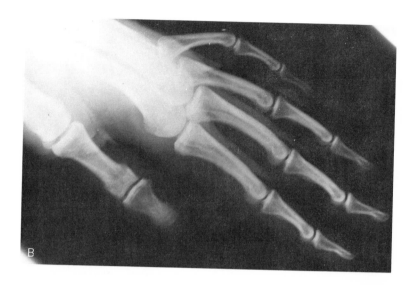

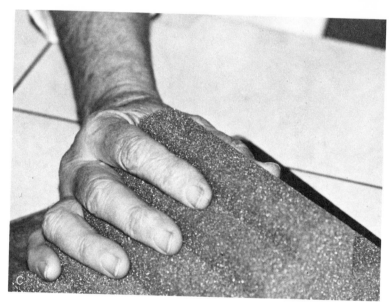

FIG. 10-3. (B) *Isolated lateral views of the digits reveal details of individual fingers. (C) A method of achieving isolated lateral views of the digits.*

splint or cast, the extremity elevated, and the patient appropriately referred. The urgency of referral depends on the problem
and each case must be assessed individually.

If a firm diagnosis cannot be made but your index of suspicion
leads you to believe that something is amiss, it is best to splint the
hand and forearm, give instructions for elevation, and arrange
specifically for a follow-up examination within 24 to 48 hours.
Advise the patient that further treatment may be necessary.

Specific Bone and Joint Injuries

Specific injuries are discussed by region, moving from the
forearm distally. Both bone and joint injuries of a given region are
discussed concurrently. Because we are dealing only with hand
injuries in this text, the discussion begins at the distal forearm
level.

DISTAL FOREARM FRACTURES

The most common distal forearm fracture is the Colles' fracture, which was described in the early nineteenth century by
Abraham Colles. In this injury the radius fractures through its
distal end and the distal fragment may tilt dorsally. With a proximal shift, some shortening and radial deviation of the hand may
occur. The ulnar styloid may or may not be fractured. The degree
of displacement and the degree of comminution vary considerably. Often the fracture is undisplaced (Fig. 10-4). Patients whose
fractures display notable shortening, displacement, or comminution in general are beyond the scope of treatment in the emergency department or office. If your consultant is nearby, the
patient should be referred at once for reduction of the fracture. If
consultation is some distance away, applying a well-padded volar
splint and giving instructions for elevation are satisfactory temporary expedients.

If the patient has a fracture considered treatable in the primary
care setting but in need of reduction, the fracture hematoma is
infiltrated with 2% lidocaine. Alternative methods of anesthesia

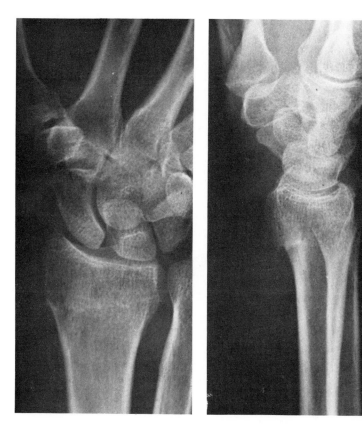

FIG. 10-4. *This minimally displaced fracture of the radius required only a cast for treatment.*

include a Bier block (intravenous lidocaine) or one of the brachial plexus blocks, but these methods are beyond the scope of the emergency department.

Reduction is accomplished by distraction of the fracture, exaggeration of the injury, and replacement of the fractured fragment. Traction with "finger traps" may make the reduction easier (Fig. 10-5). After reduction is confirmed by roentgenogram, the patient's arm is put in a well-padded long arm cast with the forearm slightly pronated. Extreme wrist positions should be avoided. The

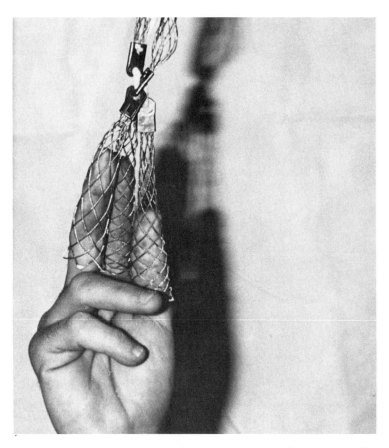

FIG. 10-5. *This device is helpful for reducing a Colles' fracture. The weight of the arm helps to relax the muscles.*

extreme Cotton-Loder position (which is ulnar deviation and wrist flexion) may result in a stiff hand. If the reduction is not easily accomplished, soft tissue may be interposed and efforts in the primary care facility should be abandoned. The patient should be referred to an appropriate consultant in this case. Following reduction the patient must keep the extremity elevated (this is aided by the long arm cast) and actively move the fingers at regular intervals (five minutes per hour) to prevent stiffness.

The obverse to Colles' fracture is Smith's fracture, with volar displacement of the fracture fragment. The principles of treatment are similar to those outlined for Colles' fracture, but reduction is done in the opposite direction.

INJURIES TO THE CARPUS

These injuries comprise a relatively small proportion of bone and joint injuries of the hand. The injury usually results from severe trauma, most often indirect force transmitted to the wrist from the hand. A history of a substantial fall or blow and a painful, tender wrist that lacks full motion should make the examiner suspect a carpal injury. Dobyns and Linsheid[3] suggest six radiographic views for accurate diagnosis: the true anteroposterior and lateral views with the wrist in a neutral position; the anteroposterior views in maximal ulnar and maximal radial deviation; and the lateral views in maximal flexion and maximal extension.

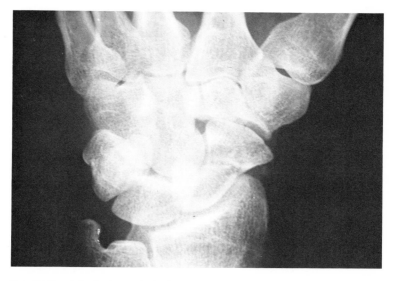

FIG. 10-6. *A typical scaphoid fracture occurred in this 44-year-old man.*

Fracture of the scaphoid bone (the carpal navicular) is by far the most common carpal injury (Fig. 10-6). Fractures may occur in several locations, but the most common is through the waist of this bone, which is near the junction of the proximal and middle thirds. The fracture may not be seen on the initial roentgenograms, and for this reason follow-up is important. If you suspect such a fracture, immobilize the patient's extremity at least in a short-arm splint. If the diagnosis can be confirmed, the patient should have a long-arm thumb spica cast. Immobilization may need to be prolonged. Nonunion of the fracture and avascular necrosis of the proximal fragment occur with some regularity even with maximal early treatment.

Dorsal chip fractures of the triquetrum bone are seen fairly often. This diagnosis can only be made with a roentgenogram, but you may suspect such an injury by finding localized tenderness. Having the patient wear a splint until tenderness subsides is all that is required.

Carpal dislocations, fracture-dislocations, subluxations, and collapse deformities occur with relative infrequency (Fig. 10-7). Most often the lunate alone or the lunate and the proximal scaphoid remain in place while the rest of the carpus dislocates dorsally. Closed reduction is frequently possible, but general or regional anesthesia is required. These are serious injuries and the patient should be referred on an urgent basis to a hand surgeon or an orthopedist.

Dobyns and Linscheid[3] classify subluxation and collapse deformities of the wrist on the basis of careful analysis and wide clinical experience. These often result from ligamentous injuries and, therefore, can be placed in the category of wrist sprains. The primary complaint would be pain and loss of wrist motion occurring either acutely or chronically. Splinting the wrist and referring the patient to a hand specialist are in order.

Fractures of the lunate are uncommon and probably result from a compression force. They may eventually result in Kienbock's disease or avascular necrosis. The roentgenographic appearance of this problem is fairly typical (Fig. 10-8). Operative treatment is indicated and the patient should be referred to a specialist.

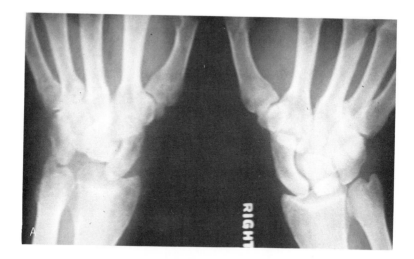

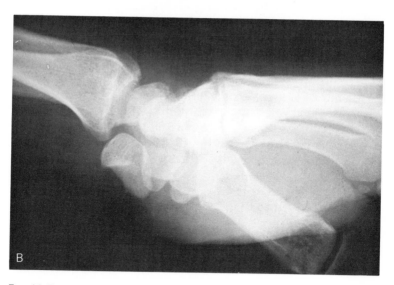

FIG. 10-7. *(A) Comparison of right and left wrists shows that a "hole"
exists where the lunate should be on the view of the left wrist. This bone
had been totally dislocated for some time when the patient was first
seen. (B) On the lateral view, the volarly dislocated lunate can be seen
clearly.*

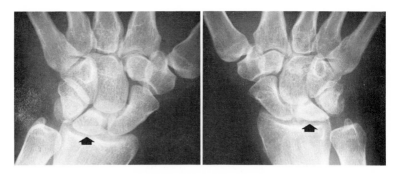

FIG. 10-8. *As a result of a fall, this young woman developed Kienbock's disease or avascular necrosis of the lunate. Arrows show the normal lunate on the left and the sclerotic one on the right.*

Other carpal fractures may be seen but they are uncommon. For these, follow the general principles of immobilization for acute injuries and the referral of patients with either acute or old injuries.

METACARPAL FRACTURES

The metacarpal bones of the fingers possess various degrees of motion that range from least in the second and third to slight in the fourth, and to some in the fifth. By contrast, the thumb metacarpal is capable of considerable motion in two planes, flexion and extension, and abduction and adduction. Shaft fractures of any of these metacarpals may cause misalignment (see Fig. 10-2B) of the digit that projects from it in either a volar-dorsal direction (angular deformity) or an ulnar-radial direction (rotary deformity). Shortening may also result from such a fracture, but this usually is not a serious problem if there is no rotary or angular deformity.

Metacarpal fractures (Figs. 10-9 and 10-10) usually heal rapidly, at least enough to allow early resumption of supervised or careful motion of the digits. Ordinarily a metacarpal fracture may be satisfactorily immobilized by applying a short-arm cast that includes the MCP joint and that of one or two of the adjacent digits. The hand should be immobilized in the position of function or close to it. An injured thumb, of course, may be immobilized by itself. After about two weeks, the fracture has usually healed enough to allow the patient to go about in a volar splint that is removed several times a day for active exercises in warm water.

If the fracture is angulated, displaced, or open, the patient should be referred for open reduction and internal fixation and debridement, if indicated. In addition to holding a fracture in an anatomic or near anatomic position, secure fixation permits early mobilization of the digits and the avoidance of a stiff hand.

Several metacarpal fractures merit individual attention, either because of their frequency or because of consequences of incorrect treatment.

INJURIES AT THE THUMB JOINT

The basal joint of the thumb is a double saddle joint that allows the metacarpal to have considerable motion in two planes. Any injury that interferes with this causes considerable loss of thumb

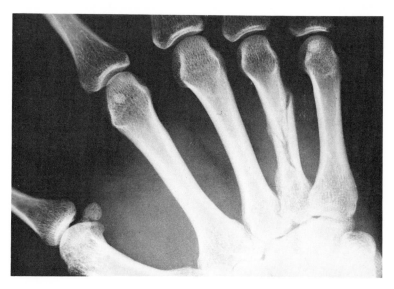

FIG. 10-9. *This oblique, comminuted, but minimally displaced metacarpal shaft fracture required immobilization but no reduction.*

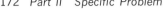

FIG. 10-10.   *This fracture of the thumb metacarpal was already two weeks old when the patient, a motorcycle police officer who had continued to work every day, was first seen for examination. Although the fracture occurred near a joint, it was a shaft fracture, not a Bennett's fracture (see Fig. 10-11).*

motion. Severe injuries may cause a dislocation of the joint or ligamentous disruption, but these are not subtle injuries and the need for referral will be obvious. Not so obvious may be a Bennett's fracture, which is an oblique fracture of the ulnar base of the thumb metacarpal that goes into the joint (Fig. 10-11). If this fracture is not reduced and held, the consequence may be an adducted thumb without good function as well as a painful joint. A Rolando fracture is a double Bennett's fracture in which two basilar fragments are intra-articular; it also should be reduced and held. Usually these fractures need to be fixed internally. Sometimes this can be done in a closed fashion and sometimes open reduction is required. All patients with such fractures should be referred to a hand surgeon or orthopedist.

INJURIES OF THE FIFTH METACARPAL

In addition to a shaft fracture like that just discussed, the fifth metacarpal may sustain a fracture at either end, which presents special problems.

The fifth metacarpal has a fair amount of mobility at both the carpometacarpal (CMC) and MCP joints. Fractures at the base or at the CMC joint, if not well reduced and held until healed, may give rise to a painful joint with loss of full mobilty and a weakened grip. Be alert for these fractures, which probably require referral of patients who sustain them to specialists. The same is true of proximal fractures of the second, third, and fourth metacarpals, but these are uncommon and usually occur only with such severe hand trauma that the need for referral is readily apparent.

Fractures of the distal end of the fifth metacarpal are common. This is the so-called boxer's fracture (Fig. 10-12), sustained by the closed fist hitting a hard object such as a wall or an opponent's jaw. The distal fragment is tilted down. Often these fractures are seen several days after they occur, no doubt because of the

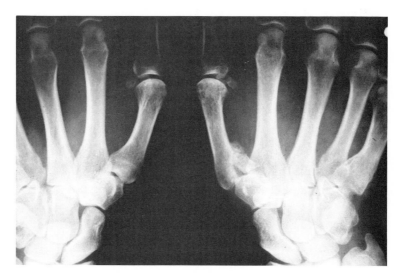

FIG. 10-11. *Comparison of right and left thumbs shows the obvious Bennett's fracture.*

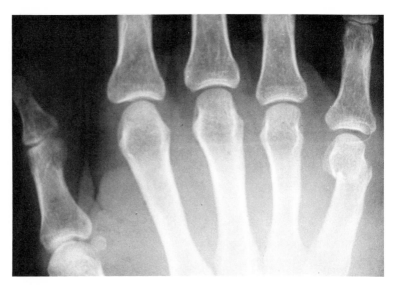

FIG. 10-12. *The typical "boxer's fracture" is a fracture of the distal end of the fifth metacarpal.*

circumstance in which they happened. If the fracture is seen near the time of injury, attempt to reduce it using an ulnar nerve block. Unless the fracture is tilted very far down, open reduction is not indicated. Even with displaced fractures, ultimate function is usually good because of the relative mobility of the metacarpal bone (Fig. 10-13). The main loss usually involves flexion of the MCP joint.

INJURIES AT THE SECOND TO FIFTH MCP JOINTS

The second through fifth metacarpophalangeal joints are similar in structure and function and may be considered together. These joints are not often subjected to isolated injury. Dislocation may occur. The involved digit will be shortened and motion at the MCP joint will be limited and painful. The diagnosis is confirmed by roentgenogram. Open reduction is often required.

Blunt trauma that occurs directly over a joint or compacting or twisting trauma may result in a painful swollen joint without actual instability. The diagnosis in such cases is traumatic synovitis, which usually subsides in several days with digit immobilization in a short-arm splint. Occasionally a cortisone injection is useful.

INJURIES AT THE THUMB MCP JOINT

The thumb MCP joint is frequently injured on its ulnar side when the collateral ligament is stretched, torn, or avulsed. This injury is popularly known as the "gamekeeper's thumb," because

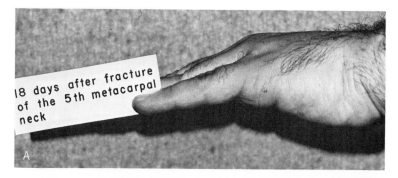

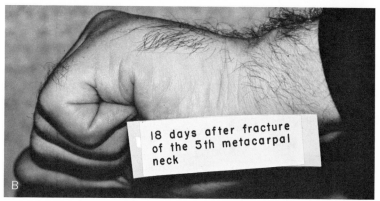

FIG. 10-13. *(A and B) Same patient as in Figure 10-12, 18 days after fracture of the fifth metacarpal neck. Function is usually excellent even when reduction is less than perfect.*

it was first described in gamekeepers[4] who sustained the chronic injury from breaking rabbits' necks. In the United States it is more commonly seen in the acute or subacute state; the variety of ways in which it occurs have as a common denominator the application of force to the proximal phalanx of the thumb to stress it in a radial direction and injure the ulnar collateral ligament. A common cause today is catching the thumb in a ski pole that has stopped abruptly while the skier keeps on moving. The diagnosis is made from the history of the mechanism of injury, the symptoms of pain and weakness with "giving away" on attempted pinch, and the signs of swelling, tenderness, and instability on the ulnar side of the joint. Stress films are useful for confirming the diagnosis (Fig. 10-14). The injury may involve an associated fracture of a portion of the proximal phalanx. Testing for instability should always be done with the joint in full extension.

If the joint is grossly unstable, the patient should be referred to a specialist for early open repair. If the tear appears to be only partial, a three-week application of a thumb spica cast may allow it to heal satisfactorily. In either situation it may be wise to have the patient seen by a hand surgeon or orthopedic surgeon.

The radial collateral ligament of the thumb may sustain the same type of injury, but it is far less common than that affecting the ulnar collateral ligament.

PROXIMAL PHALANGEAL FRACTURES

Fractures of this bone are common and may be due to direct trauma (Fig. 10-15) or indirect, twisting injuries (Fig. 10-16). If the fracture does not need reduction, or if it is easily reduced and stable upon gentle passive PIP joint motion, the injured finger and an adjacent one should be put into a short-arm splint to include the injured and one adjacent digit in the position of function or in the intrinsic plus position (MCP flexion and IP extension). At ten days to two weeks gentle active motion should be started three to four times a day if the patient is to avoid PIP stiffness. The finger should *not* be kept rigidly immobile until callus appears on the roentgenogram, because the result will be PIP stiffness that is often unalterable.

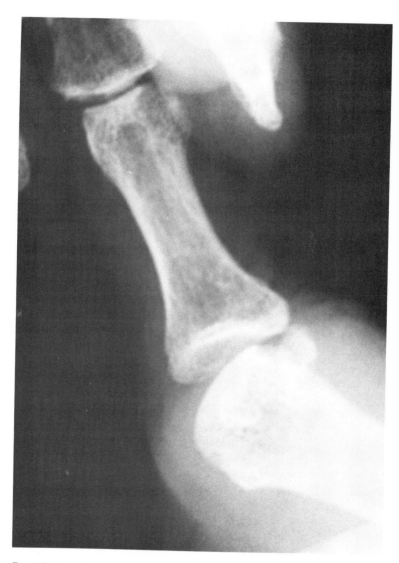

FIG. 10-14.   *The patient is a middle-aged woman who sustained a sudden force that tore the ulnar collateral ligament of the thumb, causing pain and instability. The stress roentgenogram clearly demonstrates the problem.*

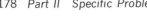

FIG. 10-15. *This 24-year-old man had an open fracture of the proximal phalanx.*

Proximal phalangeal fractures unfortunately are frequently neither easily reduced nor very stable. Even fractures that initially look stable (Fig. 10-17) may slip and create problems. I believe that many but not all proximal phalangeal fractures should be opened, reduced, and internally fixed (Fig. 10-18) to allow early resumption of PIP motion without loss of anatomic alignment.

INJURIES AT THE PIP JOINT

This little joint may be the first among equals of the joints of the hand, because its great range of motion is important to ade-

quate finger function. Significant dysfunction may be a consequence of tendon injury (see Chapter 9), fracture, or injury to a
ligament.

A relatively common and serious injury is fracture dislocation
at the PIP joint with avulsion of the volar lip of the proximal end of
the middle phalanx and dorsal dislocation of the remainder of the
middle phalanx (Fig. 10-19). This dislocation occurs because the
fracture fragment is solidly attached to the volar plate, which is
the firm fibrous structure that ordinarily prevents hyperextension
of this joint. This injury must be treated by open reduction and
internal fixation. Other fracture dislocations at the PIP joint are
less common, but in general they also require open reduction and
internal fixation.

Dislocation without fracture is also a common injury at this
joint. The injury may be closed (Figs. 10-20, 10-21) or open (Fig.

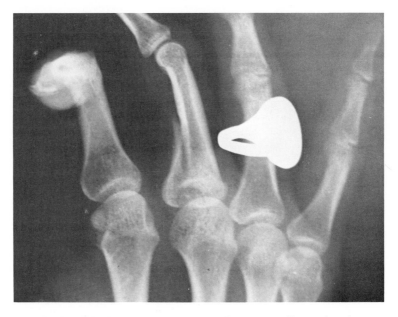

FIG. 10-16. *This 25-year-old man was "finger wrestling" when he sustained this fracture. The first step in treatment is to remove the ring. The
fracture required open reduction and internal fixation.*

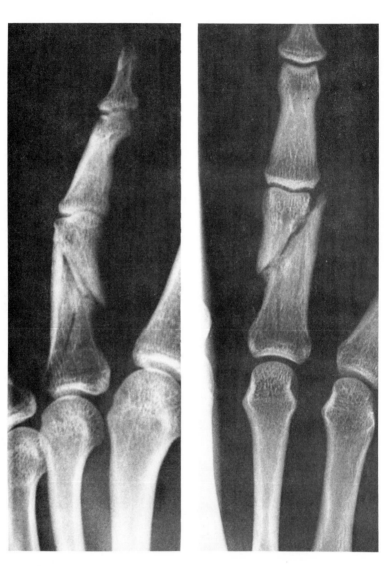

FIG. 10-17.   *This 35-year-old man had his fracture treated by four weeks of cast immobilization. The fracture had slipped a bit, but when we saw him the most serious problem was a stiff PIP joint, which could not be mobilized well.*

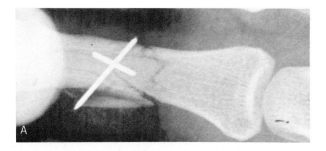

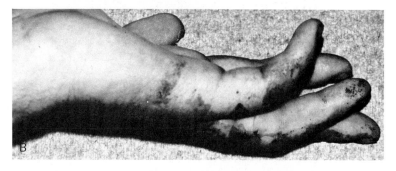

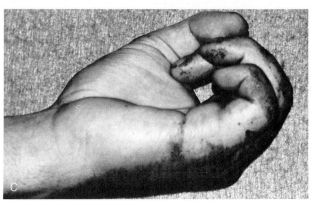

FIG. 10-18. *The same patient seen in Figure 10-15. (A) Roentgenogram taken after reduction and pin fixation of the fracture. (B) Guarded active motion was commenced seven days after fracture; this would have been impossible without internal fixation. (C) Flexing the injured ring finger. This patient had an excellent result with almost normal PIP motion.*

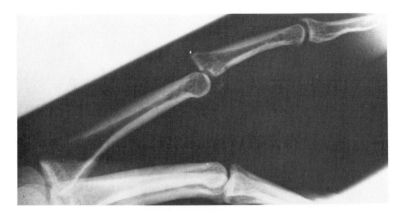

FIG. 10-19.   This type of fracture dislocation of the PIP joint always requires open reduction and fixation.

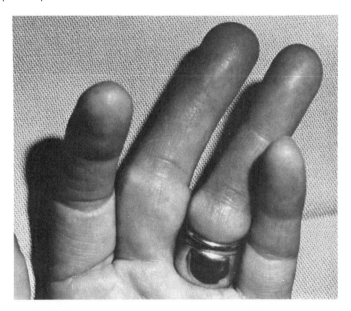

FIG. 10-20.   In this case the diagnosis of two PIP dislocations is obvious even without roentgenograms. The proximal phalangeal condyles can be seen "tenting" the volar skin, especially on the long finger. The rings on this patient's finger were difficult to remove even with a ring cutter.

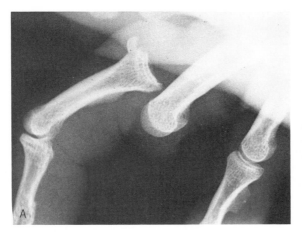

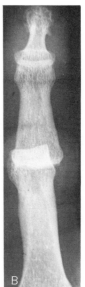

FIG. 10-21.   *Typical radiographic appearance of a PIP dislocation.*

10-22). Usually the middle phalanx dislocates dorsally. The injury merits an attempt at reduction using a finger nerve block. The diagnosis of PIP dislocation may be obvious without x-ray studies. Although roentgenograms are important, if a significant delay is anticipated, perform the reduction right away. If the joint is not easily reduced with the technique that involves traction and exaggeration of the deformity, it is not wise to persist. Failure to reduce the injury is probably due to soft tissue interposition. The patient should be referred urgently to a specialist for open reduction.

Partial dislocations of the joint may be subtle and difficult to diagnose by either physical or roentgenographic examination. Keep in mind that an adequately reduced, stable joint will go through a full range of gentle passive motion while the digit is anesthetized. If the arc of motion deviates or motion is blocked, the reduction is not adequate. In this situation, obtain roentgenograms taken in several planes and use the opposite hand for comparison.

The same general principles just discussed for the PIP joint also apply to injuries of the IP joint of the thumb.

Fig. 10-22. *Soft tissue interposition usually makes reduction of an open PIP dislocation difficult.*

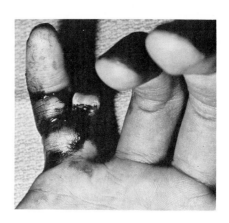

When a PIP or IP joint is adequately reduced, it should be splinted for one week, preferably in a short-arm splint in the position of function. After seven to ten days the short-arm splint is reserved for night use, and a finger splint that stabilizes just the PIP and DIP or IP joints is used during the day. The patient begins gentle active motion in warm water six to eight times per day. The splint is discarded entirely after three weeks. Early motion is critical because a stiff PIP joint is useless. For the reader interested in an in-depth discussion of joint injuries of the hand, Eaton has written an excellent short book on the subject.[5]

MIDDLE PHALANGEAL FRACTURES

The problems that arise with fractures of this bone are similar to those that accompany fractures of the proximal phalanx, but the consequences of poor treatment are slightly less serious because the distal joint is the DIP instead of the PIP. Unstable or irreducible fractures should be opened and fixed internally, especially if they are near one of the joints.

DIP JOINT INJURIES

This joint is just as subject to dislocation and fracture dislocations as the PIP joint. Dislocations may be open or closed and easy or difficult to reduce. Difficulty encountered in reduction is usually due to soft tissue interposition.

The common direction of the dislocation at this joint is volar, rather than dorsal as it is at the PIP joint. A lip of dorsal distal phalanx may break off at the insertion of the common extensor mechanism (Fig. 10-23). The remainder of the distal phalanx is pulled in a volar direction by the profundus tendon. This, of course, results in a mallet or baseball finger.

This fracture is difficult to reduce and hold by closed methods. If it involves over 30% of the joint surface, the chances of traumatic arthritis ultimately developing are substantial. Therefore, it may be wise to open, reduce, and fix the fracture. Patients may resist this much surgery at the DIP joint, and you should tell them that fusion of the joint may be done if the problem of traumatic arthritis ever becomes severe. A person loses little function with DIP fusion.

DISTAL PHALANGEAL FRACTURES

Fractures of this little bone are usually due to crushing or ripping injuries that inflict substantial soft tissue trauma. Care of the soft tissue injury takes precedence, and the fracture can generally be molded and held in place with the soft tissue repair. If the bone does not become infected, pain-free healing usually takes place (Fig. 10-24).

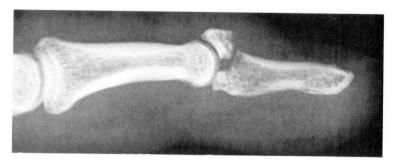

FIG. 10-23. *Fracture dislocation of the DIP joint may cause mallet finger deformity, which is why patients with this deformity should have a radiographic study.*

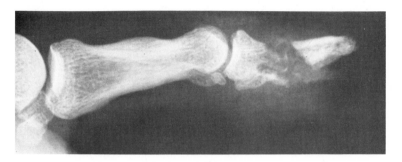

FIG. 10-24.   *Typical shaft fracture of the distal phalanx. Fractures of the distal tuft are even more common.*

Desmitis of the Upper Extremity

The term *desmitis* derives from the Greek word *desmos* or band. The upper extremity has many bands or ligamentous structures. Some of these structures are easily definable and injuries to them are equally definable. Other structures are less well-defined but prone to soreness, tenderness, and general misery.

Probably the best known of these desmitides is *lateral epicondylitis*, or tennis elbow. This condition commences with either indirect stress or a direct blow. All of the extrinsic extensors arise at or near the lateral epicondyle. This means that in persons with lateral epicondylitis, the use of the hand in any position may cause pain depending on whether the wrist or finger extensors are in use (see Synergism in Chapter 1). Diagnosis is made by eliciting tenderness with direct palpation or by causing pain with wrist extension against force.

Lateral epicondylitis is usually self-limited if the causative stress is removed. An injection of a long-acting cortisone preparation and lidocaine into the point of maximal pain and tenderness may be efficacious in relieving the symptoms. A cock-up wrist splint relieves stress on the wrist extensors and is often helpful. A Velcro-fastened strap placed on the upper forearm just below the lateral epicondyle may help give relief. If none of these conservative measures succeed, the patient may need to be referred for consideration for one of several surgical approaches to the problem, none of which are guaranteed. *Medial epicondylitis* is similar, except that the flexor tendons are affected. Treatment approaches are similar.

Misery about the wrist, especially on the ulnar side, may fall into the same category of desmitis, but identifiable problems should be ruled out. The treatment approaches are the same: immobilization, administration of cortisone or anti-inflammatory medication, and possibly ultrasound treatments.

Other conditions probably akin to these desmitides include DeQuervain's disease (Chapter 9) and carpal tunnel syndrome (Chapter 14). It is my observation that many of these problems occur and persist in people who have jobs that require the hand to perform tasks more arduous than those to which it is suited. A change of jobs may be required, but the patient may resist this because arduous jobs are often more remunerative than lighter work. This may create an impasse between doctor, patient, worker's compensation insurance company, and employer. A patient in this predicament will probably have been referred for one or more consultations by the time the problem progresses very far. Usually the solution is some type of compromise that leaves none of the parties happy.

REFERENCES

1. *California Work Injuries.* Department of Industrial Relations, State of California, 1974.

2. Kilgore, E. S., Jr., et al.: Post-traumatic trapped dislocations of the proximal interphalangeal joint. J. Trauma, *16*:481–487, 1976.

3. Dobyns, J. H., and Linscheid, R. L.: Fractures and dislocations of the wrist. *In* Rockwood, C. A., and Green, D. P. (eds.): Fractures. Philadelphia, J. B. Lippincott, 1975.

4. Campbell, C. S.: Gamekeeper's thumb. J. Bone Joint Surg., *37B*:148–149, 1955.

5. Eaton, R. G.: Joint Injuries of the Hand. Springfield, Ill., Charles C Thomas, 1971.

11

Burns and Other Injuries Due to Nonmechanical Force

Most injuries are caused by mechanical force; the injuries discussed in this chapter are caused primarily by non-mechanical force. The results of nonmechanical energy expenditure can be awesome to behold. Thermal, chemical, and electrical energy damage or destroy living cells by denaturing protein. Cold damages or destroys cells by causing intracellular crystal formation and dehydration. As a general rule, but not absolutely, skin is the primary tissue system injured, with deep tissues being damaged secondarily, often by exposure.

Emergency and other primary care physicians see many of these injuries only in passing, because they are often severe enough not only for hospital admission but referral to specialized treatment centers or burn units. A prompt recognition of these potentially serious injuries and vigorous early initiation of treatment may prevent much subsequent misery and disability.

Burns of the Hand

These injuries forcibly remind us that the acceptable temperature milieu for living creatures is rather narrow. The hands are especially susceptible to injuries at either extreme of temperature because of their exposed position.

Most burns or thermal injuries are caused by fire. However, serious burns may also occur as a consequence of direct contact with hot objects or immersion in hot liquids. Friction injuries, which are sometimes classified with burns, have been placed with complex injuries in Chapter 12.

Burns are different from other injuries with which this text has dealt. With a burn, skin is selectively destroyed, and one can then appreciate what a marvelous and versatile organ it is. The skin, the largest organ in humans, protects and preserves the internal environment of the body. In general terms this function allows the organism to live and function. In specific terms, this protected internal environment allows the finely aligned joints of the hand to be moved through a full range of motion by intrinsic and extrinsic musculotendinous units without difficulty. This homeostatic situation is abruptly changed by a burn. Even a "trivial" burn results in some swelling and interference with the normal range of motion of the hand. If the burn penetrates through skin to fat, fascia, and tendons, a permanent alteration may take place, and result in a hand that is barely recognizable as such (Fig. 11-1).

A burn should be neither underestimated nor undertreated. With careful management, a fairly deep burn may heal completely with no residual impairment. With careless management, a superficial burn may be converted to a deeper injury as a consequence of infection and may heal with significant scar formation and loss of hand motion.

ASSESSMENT OF BURN DEPTH

This assessment is easy to define on paper and often difficult to accurately gauge in practice. The classic three categories of burns are first, second, and third degree. A *first degree burn* involves only enough of the epidermis to produce erythema; usually, it is not difficult to be accurate in assessing this burn. *Second degree burns* are intermediate in severity, running the gamut from being almost like a first degree burn to almost like a third degree burn. The essence of treatment of a second degree burn is to manage it according to whichever extreme it most resembles,

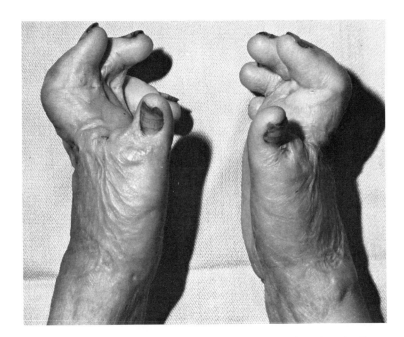

FIG. 11-1. *The hands of a three-year-old boy who suffered major flame burns four months previously. Severe contractions developed despite early vigorous treatment. The hands were made functional over the following four years by using surgical procedures, splinting, and compression.*

the first or third degree. The usual sign of a second degree burn is the formation of one or more blisters (Fig. 11-2). Second degree burns are probably more accurately classified as superficial partial-thickness or deep partial-thickness burns.

In third degree burns, the epidermis, its deep appendages (the sweat glands and hair follicles), and the dermis are destroyed. The skin is characteristically charred and insensitive (Fig. 11-3). It may be difficult to distinguish this burn from a deep partial-thickness (second degree) burn. Patients with both deep second and third degree burns should be referred for definitive care, even if the burned area is fairly small. This is especially true if hands, feet, face, or genitalia are involved.

TREATMENT OF BURNS

The immediate treatment of a thermal injury is obviously governed by both the extent and depth of the injury.[1] The discussion here is limited to burns of the hand and forearm, which by themselves would seldom cause severe prostration and shock. A patient who has burns extending beyond these areas might require life-resuscitative measures, which would be started at once.

As with any injury, control of panic and pain are first steps. With many burns, the application of running cold water or immersion in iced water does much to alleviate pain and prevent further damage. Analgesics may be necessary, but it is wise to avoid oversedating a patient before a medical history can be taken and

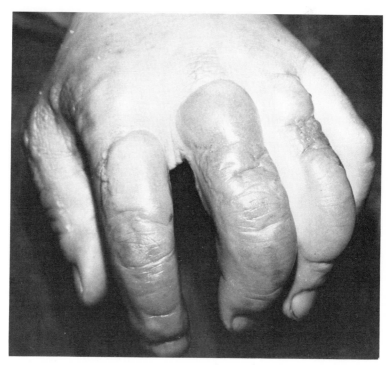

FIG. 11-2.   *A 50-year-old man sustained typical partial-thickness burns when his cigarette lighter flared up.*

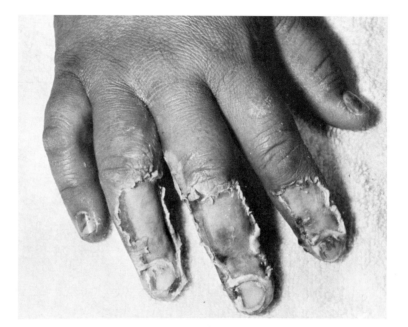

FIG. 11-3. *A 40-year-old lady caught three fingers in a hot presser at a laundry, which caused full-thickness (third degree) burns.*

the injury evaluated adequately. If one administers a large dose of morphine or meperidine and the injury then appears to be compatible with outpatient care, the effect of the analgesic may cause more harm than the injury itself.

The next step is to clean the wound gently with a cold, mild, antiseptic solution. The physician should perform this step, because it is an ideal time to assess the extent and depth of the burn.

First degree or superficial partial-thickness burns of the hand (mild second degree burns) should be dressed with nonadherent gauze (Xeroform), 4-in. × 4-in. sterile gauze, foam sponge (Reston) and an appropriate plaster splint to keep the extremity in the position of function. Elevate to heart level or higher with an appropriate sling (see Chapter 4), give a prescription for analgesics, make provision for follow-up examination in a day or two.

If extensive blistering has been caused by the burn, leave the blisters intact if possible. Reepithelialization occurs more rapidly in a moist, noninfected environment, and intact blisters provide this environment. By the time the blisters finally collapse, healing will be almost complete beneath them (Fig. 11-4). If the blisters have already broken when the patient is first seen, an open wound exists. Loose debris should be carefully cleared away using sterile techniques.

Various dressing techniques for open or closed partial-thickness burns are acceptable. I favor the use of silver sulfadiazine cream (Silvadene) applied generously over the burn wound, which is then dressed occlusively and appropriately splinted. This dressing must be changed every day. The therapeutic value of Silva-

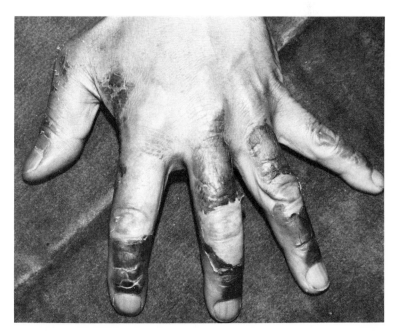

FIG. 11-4. *Patient shown in Figure 11-2 after two weeks of treatment with silver sulfadiazine cream and splinting. The dark scaly skin resulted from the silver. Note the absence of swelling. Function was almost completely restored at this point.*

dene may be lost if the dressings are not changed at least once a day and the Silvadene reapplied. If daily dressing changes are not possible, it is probably better to apply zinc oxide and cover the wound with nonadherent gauze.

The burned hand must be handled gently. Prevention of swelling and contamination is critical if infection and deepening of the burn injury are to be avoided. Appropriate tetanus prophylaxis should be administered.

Deep partial-thickness burns are often difficult to distinguish from full-thickness burns. The usual test of sensibility (second degree burn) versus no sensibility (third degree burn) may not be helpful. Both may look like tanned leather. A patient with a burn of this severity should probably be referred on an urgent basis to a hand surgeon or a surgeon with an interest and expertise in burns. If consultative help is not readily available, admit the patient to the hospital and dress the hand with Silvadene (silver sulfadiazine), splint it, and elevate it. If the hand and forearm become tight and choked owing to swelling under unyielding eschar, it may become mandatory to perform an escharotomy (Fig. 11-5). With third degree burns with loss of sensibility,

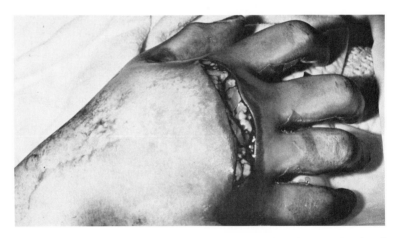

Fɪɢ. 11-5. *Third degree burns of the hand. The patient has a "claw hand in disguise," caused by dorsal swelling which forces the MCP joints into hyperextension. This constriction must be released by escharotomy.*

escharotomy may be performed without anesthesia, but an appropriate sterile field is required. Incision is made until the constriction is relieved when normal or nearly normal tissue is reached, usually at the subcutaneous level. The lines of incision suggested in Chapter 5 may be followed.

Deep partial-thickness and full-thickness burns often require excision of the burned tissue down to the subcutaneous area, followed by application of a graft (Fig. 11-6). Although deep partial-thickness areas will heal without a graft, the scarring may be so intense that the hand is rendered useless by virtue of loss of motion. Scar formation tends to be excessive in children. It is not wise to persist in managing a burn that does not show progressive healing by 10 to 14 days; such patients should be referred to the appropriate specialists.

AREA OF BURN

Most thermal injuries occur on the dorsal part of the hand, especially because it is a natural reaction to shield the face when flames are pressing in. For reasons previously enumerated, the dorsum of the hand is less able to tolerate a burn injury, because of its relatively thinner skin as compared to the palm. Dorsal skin is also elastic, and loss of elasticity due first to edema and then to scar formation means loss of hand function.

By contrast, palmar skin is much thicker than dorsal skin and much less elastic. This means that the injuring agent usually must be more intense to cause a significant injury. Principles of treatment are the same for both dorsal and volar wounds, but bear in mind that the margin for error is less when managing burns on the dorsum.

SOME SPECIFIC BURNS

A few specific types of burn wounds merit individual mention. *Hot tar burns* are encountered occasionally in roofers. The patient appears with all or part of the hand covered with tar, which is cool by the time the patient is seen. If the tar cover is extensive, the patient should be admitted to the hospital. Avoid the temptation

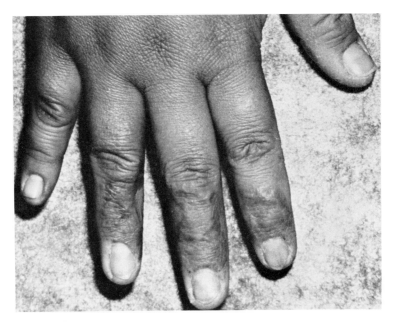

FIG. 11-6.   *The patient shown in Figure 11-3 had eschar excision followed by split-thickness skin grafting. Healing was rapid and function remains excellent.*

to remove the tar with vigorous mechanical means, because you may further damage the burned skin. Ashbell et al.[2] have demonstrated that petrolatum-based ointments, such as Neosporin, applied hourly will slowly dissolve the tar without trauma. As the tar separates, the underlying burn can be treated by the usual appropriate measures.

Circumferential hot water burns in children should be a signal that child abuse has been perpetrated by holding the extremity in hot water. Be especially concerned about choked tissues with this type of burn, because there is no area for "give" as the tissue swells. The need for escharotomy is likely in this situation.

Compression burns occur as a consequence of catching part or all of the hand in a mechanical ironer, press, or roller. The burn wound is straightforward, but be aware of possible damage to other tissues such as a fracture due to the compressive force.

Cold Injury

Cold injury occurs with adequate exposure of parts to a cold environment. Wetness can decrease the exposure time necessary for injury, as can direct contact with cold metal. The injuries vary in severity from trivial to fatal tissue destruction. Cold injuries are classified much like burn injuries: superficial (first degree); partial-thickness injury characterized by blister formation (second degree); full-thickness injury with gangrene and skin loss (third degree); total loss of the part (fourth degree).[3]

Emergency treatment of these injuries depends on their severity. The critical step in treatment is rapid rewarming of the injured part in water heated between 40° and 42°C. Water temperatures higher than this may be harmful, and lower temperatures will not provide maximal benefit. Heavy sedation may be required during the rewarming.[3]

Management of these injuries following rewarming is similar to that for burn injuries and meticulous wound care, splinting, elevation and administration of analgesics. Patients with medium to deep partial-thickness injuries or greater injuries should be hospitalized and consultation sought.

Sympathectomy, either by surgical[4] or pharmacologic means,[5] has been advocated by some for the treatment of these injuries, but its role has not been clearly established. It causes vasodilatation.

Even if the patient comes through the cold injury episode without loss of digits, he or she may be far more susceptible to repeated injury from cold and should be warned about this possibility.

Chemical Injuries

In general, these injuries are far less common than thermal injuries but they may be seen with some frequency in certain areas where the presence of a specific industry increases the risk of exposure to certain chemicals. The injuries may be classified as acid, due to the hydrogen ion (H^+) or alkali, due to the hydroxyl ion (OH^-). These ions may persist in destroying tissue until they are neutralized by copious water irrigation.[6] In other words, the injury (often referred to as a chemical burn) may still be progressing when the patient is first seen. Acids produce coagulation necrosis, and alkalis produce liquefaction necrosis. Apparently the hydroxyl ion may be passed from molecule to molecule causing successive cells to be denatured before it is finally inactivated. By contrast, acid is believed to be neutralized on initial contact.

In general, acid burns are treated with copious water irrigation, which may be followed by irrigation with dilute sodium bicarbonate. If the injuring agent is a phenol (carbolic acid), neutralization with ethyl alcohol is recommended.

The most troublesome and painful acid burn is caused by hydrofluoric acid.[7,8] This is one of the more common acid burns. Among other uses, it is employed by makers of stained glass windows, and this is an increasingly popular avocational pursuit. The acid penetrates the skin and causes exquisitely painful lesions. The first emergency step is to irrigate the wound with large amounts of water. The injection of 10% calcium gluconate beneath the eschar after establishing suitable regional anesthesia has been advocated. Soaking the injury with Hyamine #1622 (a high-molecular-weight quaternary ammonium compound) may offer relief. Benzalkonium chloride (Zephiran) can be used if Hyamine is not available. Because of the penetration of the acid, debridement of nails and skin may be necessary to be certain that acid is not trapped in tissue.

Alkali burns should be treated with copious water irrigation, followed by irrigation with 0.5% to 5.0% acetic acid as a neutralizing solution. Because of the penetration potential of alkalis, the irrigation should continue for some time to ensure neutralization. Remember that cement can cause a severe alkali burn.[9]

For an excellent discussion of chemical burns with considerable detail about specific burns (including phosphorus burns), I refer you to the paper by Orcutt and Pruitt.[10]

Electrical Injury

Fortunately, electrical injuries are uncommon. The physician should distinguish between electrical injuries caused by "domestic'' low-voltage electricity, which usually lies in the 100-volt range, and high-tension electrical injury.[11] Low-voltage injuries usually cause local scorching with some necrosis but generally do not spread along tissue planes or cause serious systemic effects.

By contrast, high-tension electrical injuries due to currents of 500 volts and more cause severe local and systemic injury. The current travels along the path of least resistance, namely through the nerves and vessels. The overlying skin initially may appear normal, and the only clue to the current's direction is the charred area where it exits from the body, either to a ground or sometimes to another part of the body, as when it arcs across the axilla.

Tissue destruction along the course of the current is extensive, and loss of all or part of a limb is not uncommon. Severe systemic effects also appear in the cardiac, renal, gastrointestinal, and central nervous systems.[12] Any patient who appears to have a high-tension electrical injury should be immediately hospitalized and closely observed.

REFERENCES

1. Newmeyer, W. L., and Kilgore, E. S., Jr.: Management of the burned hand. Phys. Ther., *57*:16–23, 1977.

2. Ashbell, T. S., et al: Tar and grease removal from injured parts. Plast. Reconstr. Surg., *40*:330–331, 1967.

3. Hermann, G., et al.: The problem of frostbite in civilian medical practice. Surg. Clin. North Am., *43*:519–536, 1936.

4. Golding, M., et al.: The role of sympathectomy in frostbite, with a review of 68 cases. Surgery, *57*:774–777, 1965.

5. Porter, J. M., et al.: Intra-arterial sympathetic blockade in the treatment of clinical frostbite. Am. J. Surg., *132*:625–630, 1976.

6. Currevi, P. W., et al.: The treatment of chemical burns. Specialized diagnostic, therapeutic, and prognostic considerations. J. Trauma, *10*:634–642, 1970.

7. Dibbell, D. G., et al.: Hydrofluoric acid burns of the hand. J. Bone Joint Surg., *52A*:931–936, 1970.

8. Reinhardt, C. F., et al.: Hydrofluoric acid burn treatment. Am. Indust. Hyg. Assoc. J., *27*:166–171, 1966.

9. Meherin, J. M., and Schomaker, T. P.: The cement burn: Its etiology, pathology and treatment. JAMA, *112*:1322–1326, 1939.

10. Orcutt, T. J., and Pruitt, B. A.: Chemical injuries of the upper extremity. *In* Salisbury, R. E., and Pruitt, B. A. (eds.): Burns of the Upper Extremity. (Vol. XIX, Major Problems in Clinical Surgery, ed. by J. E. Dumphy and P. E. Ebert) Philadelphia, W. B. Saunders, 1976.

11. Brown, H. G.: Electrical and cold injuries of the hand. Orthop. Clin. North Am. *1*:321–323, 1970.

12. DiVincenti, F. C., et al.: Electrical injuries. A review of 65 cases. J. Trauma, 9:497–507, 1969.

Complex Injuries

C OMPLEX injury was defined in an earlier chapter as an injury in which at least one tissue system has sustained a serious injury in addition to the skin, or in which the loss of skin is so extensive that a major skin graft or pedicle is necessary for treatment. Certain complex injuries to tissue systems (such as nerves, tendons, bones and joints) and certain types of complex injuries (such as burns, electrical and chemical injuries, and amputation) have warranted individual discussions. Into this chapter fall all the other complex injuries that cannot be neatly categorized by tissue system or wounding agent. Their only common denominator is that several tissue systems have been damaged or may become damaged. In the first type of injury, the emphasis is placed on correct early management, while in the second type the emphasis is on recognition of potential problems and diagnosis with correct early management following as a logical consequence.

General Management of Complex Injuries

These injuries are usually open. The mechanisms of injury are legion, but have in common great mechanical force. These are the mangling, crushing, or tearing injuries of high-speed machinery; the blasting, ripping injuries of bullets (Fig. 12-1); and the crushing, grinding injuries of heavy objects (Fig. 12-2). The skin has been torn, tendons have been ripped or demolished, nerves may have been destroyed entirely, bones and joints have been broken and smashed.

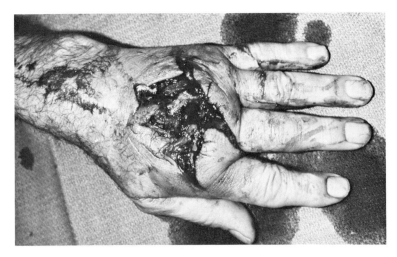

FIG. 12-1.   *This 50-year-old man was inspecting a loaded pistol that was accidentally fired. The palmar entrance wound was much smaller than this large exit wound (see Fig. 12-4).*

IMMEDIATE CARE

The immediate concern of the treating physician is to establish control of the situation. Pain, panic, and hemorrhage must be controlled. The need for hospitalization is obvious whether it be at the receiving institution or another facility. A quick assessment of the wound following the usual sequence is useful, but actual probing of the wound should be minimized or skipped altogether. The entire extremity should be freed of all encumbrances as expeditiously as possible. The injured extremity should be supported, elevated to heart level, and dressed in a bulky compressive dressing using sterile technique.

The establishment of an intravenous line in the uninjured extremity is the next step. Pain should be controlled with an appropriate analgesic, but the patient should not be sedated so heavily that he or she can no longer respond to questioning. In such a situation, the intravenous administration of cephalosporin is the ideal antibiotic therapy. Tetanus immune globulin or teta-

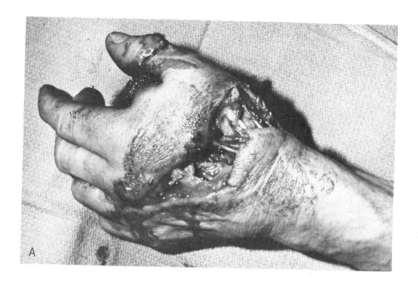

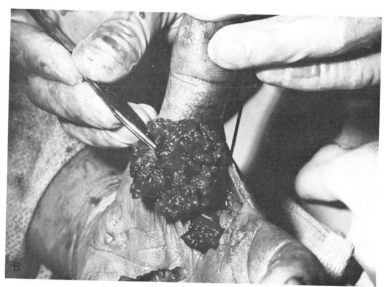

FIG. 12-2. (A) A 35-year-old man caught his hand in a powerful electric winch at a shipyard. (B) The adductor pollicis was extruded like toothpaste from a tube.

nus toxoid should be administered in accordance with the patient's history of immunization. Note any pertinent medical or drug history.

Sometimes hemorrhage can be a problem with injuries of this type. If it cannot be controlled with the bulky compressive dressing and elevation (even holding the extremity maximally over the patient's head), a tourniquet may be required; this should be set up as described in Chapter 3. A tourniquet is usually needed for only a few minutes to stop bleeding. Generally one is not needed at all.

A roentgenogram is usually a necessity in injuries of this sort. As soon as the immediate situation is under control and a blood sample has been drawn and sent for appropriate laboratory studies, the patient should be taken to the radiology department for views of the extremity. At the same time a preoperative chest film may be taken. Remember, do not accept a verbal or written radiology report; it is mandatory that the examining physician review the films. Preferably these films should be kept with the patient so that they are available in the operating room.

At this point, the patient may be either returned to the emergency department holding ward or admitted pending a call from surgery. An electrocardiogram can now be obtained if indicated. The patient, of course, has been kept NPO since arrival in the emergency department. This small point cannot be emphasized too strongly, as well-meaning but ill-informed friends or relatives may give the patient a drink, or an uncooperative patient may just ignore the injunction not to eat or drink. The patient is now ready for surgery or transfer.

PRINCIPLES OF OPERATIVE TREATMENT

The management of certain complex injuries is presented here for those primary care physicians who do not have a consultant readily available for referral and therefore may be required to perform certain basic operative steps.

Evaluation of the complex injury proceeds under regional or general anesthetic. A cuff connected to a pneumatic tourniquet should be in place. You may either elevate the arm for one minute and inflate the cuff or start the procedure without the cuff in-flated. With a badly mangled hand, compressively wrapping the arm prior to inflation of the pneumatic cuff should not be done.

Start irrigation with Ringer's lactate or normal saline when the anesthesiologist indicates that the patient is ready. If you wish, bacitracin or another antibiotic may be added to the irrigating solution. Irrigation may be done with bulb syringes or a mechanical irrigator. The purpose of the irrigation is to remove loose debris, such as separated tissue, blood clots, and pieces of foreign material. In conjunction with irrigation, obvious loose tissue and especially foreign material can be mechanically removed. Be careful about removing ground-in dirt. Do not traumatize tissue severely just to make certain that every speck of dirt has been removed. This will only serve to enhance tissue swelling and reduce vascular perfusion that is already marginal.

After irrigation and removal of loose material, carefully debride obviously devitalized but attached tissue. Always err on the side of removing too little rather than too much: you can always take out more tissue, but you cannot put tissue back. Sometimes debridement is easier to perform with the tourniquet deflated, because vascularity provides a clue to viability. During this phase of the procedure, any obvious bleeding vessels are clamped and tied with fine nylon or cauterized.

If the operator is sufficiently experienced, two further steps should be performed: skeletal stabilization and wound coverage. Skeletal stabilization may be simple and merely involve reduction of a fracture or dislocation, or it may be complex, as in the case of significant bone loss. Some type of wire fixation, by Kirschner or Concept wires or their equivalent, is often required. Each situation must be individually evaluated and treated.

The ideal wound cover is local skin. If local skin has been lost in the injury process and a widely gaping wound remains, there are two choices for covering the wound: (1) leave the wound open and cover it with nonadherent gauze or gauze impregnated with an antiseptic solution (but avoid any solution that is caustic or injurious to open tissues); (2) cover the wound with a split-thickness skin graft. A split-thickness graft in this situation provides a biologic dressing rather than definitive treatment. A thin graft of

$^{10}/_{1000}$ to $^{12}/_{1000}$ of an inch is the proper thickness. For ease of application it may be harvested and laid *outside* down on non-adherent gauze that has been precut to the approximate size of the wound. The graft-gauze composite is then laid in the wound and molded to get into all the nooks and crannies. The graft may be held in place by packing wet cotton or wet gauze to fit it into the contours of the wound. This bolus can be held in place with porous adhesive paper strips (Steri-Strips) or foam sponge (Reston). Remember, this is only a biologic dressing. If it is available, porcine skin would serve well as a dressing in this situation.

The hand is then dressed as described in Chapter 4. As has been emphasized repeatedly, swelling must be prevented so that vascular perfusion will be adequate. This does more to prevent infection and aid ultimate function than administration of all the antibiotics known. Elevate the injured part to heart level or above at all times. Be wary about suspending the hand from an intravenous pole unless the elbow is supported at all times. If the hand is elevated without elbow support, the suspending rope or strap forms a noose at the wrist and chokes off dorsal venous and lymphatic drainage.

Following this basic operative management of the patient with a mangled or crushed hand, the patient should remain hospitalized in an appropriate facility where further definitive care can be delivered if necessary. (This may entail transfer to another institution by suitable means of transportation.) Further surgery may be necessary early, especially if skeletal injury requires internal fixation or major skin loss needs pedicle flap coverage.

Specific Open Injuries

The foregoing procedures should serve well in the initial treatment of all of these open complex injuries. As emphasized, attention is directed to the management of the wound and to making certain that healing occurs early and free of complications so that reconstructive surgery as necessary can be undertaken without undue delay. Some specific injuries are attended by characteristic problems that merit consideration.

HIGH-SPEED MACHINERY INJURIES

Two kinds of injury occur in these instances: first is the injury done at the point of impact with attendant damage to all tissue; second is the indirect injury caused by the driving or rotational force of the machinery pulling or tearing long structures such as nerves or musculotendinous units. It is not unusual for a tendon to be grabbed at its distal end and avulsed all the way to the musculotendinous junction (Fig. 12-3). Joints remote from the impact area may be dislocated, and bones remote from the impact area may be fractured. It is always important to examine the entire upper extremity and order all appropriate roentgenographic views.

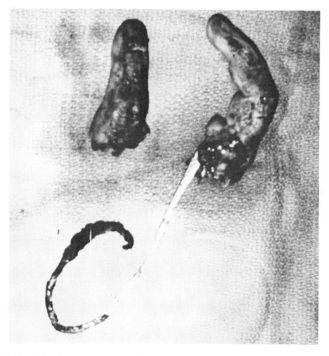

FIG. 12-3. *The fingers of a stationary engineer who caught his hand in a generator flywheel. The entire profundus tendon was yanked out to a point near the musculotendinous junction.*

GUNSHOT WOUNDS

Fortunately most civilian gunshot wounds result from low-velocity missiles. Most "civilian" guns are low-muzzle-velocity weapons (under 1000 feet per second), while military rifles such as the M-16 model produce muzzle velocities that exceed 2000 feet per second. No one who has witnessed the results of a high-velocity missile has failed to be impressed by the damage of the blast effect, which occurs remote from the wound. The wound of entrance of a bullet (Fig. 12-4A) may be small while the wound of exit (Fig. 12-1) is much larger. A corresponding cone-shaped area of injury expands from the entrance to the exit. Soft tissue structures such as tendons and nerves are often physically intact after a gunshot wound, while bones and joints are demolished (Fig. 12-4B).

CRUSH AND COMPRESSION WOUNDS

Obviously an element of crush and compression forces occurs with high-speed machinery injuries, but the indirect violence may be even greater. However, with strict crush injuries the local damage may be much greater but damage remote from the impact area is less likely to occur. Local wound contamination is likely to be greater with this type of injury (Fig. 12-5).

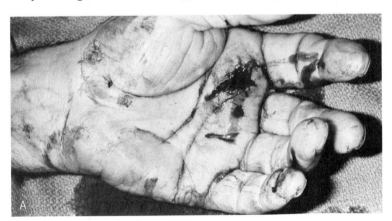

FIG. 12-4. (A) *Volar surface of the hand shown in Figure 12-1.*

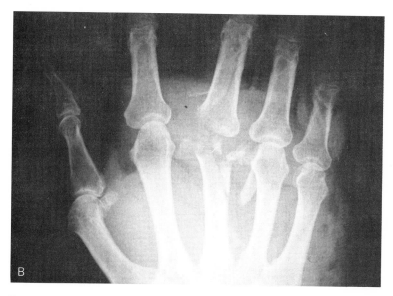

FIG. 12-4.   (B) Roentgenogram showing that the third MCP joint was destroyed.

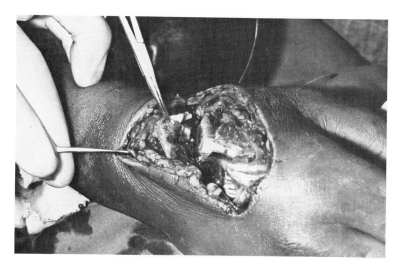

FIG. 12-5.   Ax wound of the dorsal proximal hand.

A wound akin to this type but meriting a separate category is the *friction avulsing injury* (Fig. 12-6), in which a large area of skin is torn away along with some or all of the underlying structures. This is a situation for debridement and immediate split-thickness skin grafting rather than the immediate use of a pedicle flap. I firmly believe that large pedicle flaps are to be avoided in an acute situation. Little is to be gained by this technique and much can be lost.

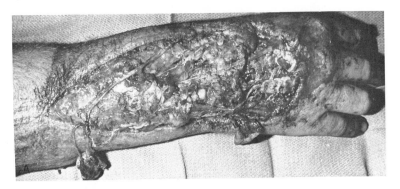

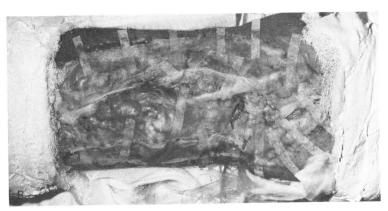

Fɪɢ. 12-6. (A) *This man was in a car that overturned and his dorsal hand and forearm were dragged along the highway causing this devastating injury. (B) Six days after injury and two days after application of a split thickness skin graft to close the wound. Eventually, pedicle coverage was required.*

Potential Injuries

Potential is perhaps not a broad-enough term to accurately describe these injuries, which may be either potential or unrecognized. As the time-honored aphorism so succinctly states, "Chance favors the prepared mind"; so it is with diagnosis of certain potentially devastating injuries.

HIGH-PRESSURE INJECTION INJURY

At first view (Fig. 12-7A) this injury appears to be the most benign and innocuous of all. The clue to its deadliness lies in the mechanism of injury. The patient recounts that he or she was using a high-pressure grease gun or paint gun when it accidentally

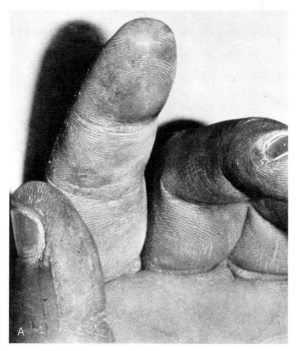

FIG. 12-7. (A) *This patient was cleaning a paint gun when it accidentally discharged into his index finger.*

penetrated a distal volar finger or other area. The patient will often be uncertain about how much material escaped into the hand, and won't be in much pain if seen soon after the injury.

The substance in the high-pressure gun, once it has penetrated the skin, follows the tissue plane of least resistance. In the finger, this is usually the flexor tendon sheath. Damage is inflicted by pressure, possibly by the toxicity of the injected substance, and possibly by heat if the substance was hot. This constitutes an absolute surgical emergency. The patient should be taken to the operating room without delay and the finger opened widely, extending the incision into the palm (Fig. 12-7B). As much of the substance as possible should be mechanically removed. A thor-

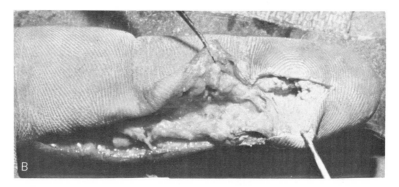

Fig. 12-7.   *(B) An immediate wide decompression was done.*

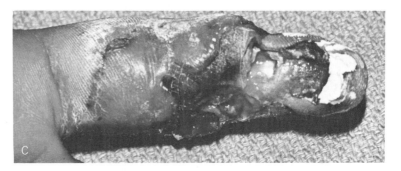

Fig. 12-7.   *(C) Within two weeks, the finger looked like this.*

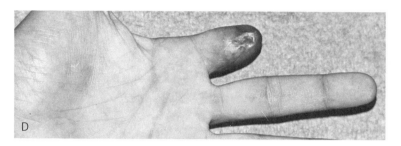

FIG. 12-7. (D) *Eventually PIP disarticulation of the finger was required.*

ough irrigation should be performed, and the wound should be left open. Even with this treatment, the finger may be lost (Fig. 12-7 C and D).

COMPARTMENT SYNDROMES

Trauma of various types may cause arterial injury, subfascial edema, or hematoma and consequent ischemia of muscles and nerves. In its ultimate stage, this is known as Volkmann's ischemic contracture, the classic cause of which is supracondylar humeral fracture in children. As the fracture is reduced, the radial pulse disappears, the forearm becomes hard and painful, and sensibility in the hand disappears. This syndrome is due to a direct injury of the brachial artery or to reflex arterial spasm.

Less well-recognized is that this complex of symptoms may be initiated by soft tissue injury[1] in the absence of a fracture. It may follow an acute severe compression, such as that caused by industrial rollers, or prolonged compression. The latter situation typically occurs in drug overdose patients who lie on their forearms for prolonged periods of time. Penetrating forearm injuries may cause a significant hematoma formation, which puts intense pressure in the forearm compartment and causes the syndrome.

Whether a compartment syndrome results from a brachial artery injury or from a direct forearm injury, capillary permeability increases and compromises intimate muscle circulation. Unless the pressure is relieved, myonecrosis and neuronecrosis with contracture and loss of sensibility will follow.

Be especially aware of the possibility of this syndrome in patients who come into emergency departments with drug overdoses. If the patient is conscious, the symptoms are initial intense pain followed by a loss of sensibility.

The most consistently reliable sign is the presence of a rock-hard forearm with progressive flexion contracture of the digits. As the syndrome progresses, the digits can be straightened only with increasing force. The syndrome occurs in the presence or absence of the radial pulse.

Any patient with forearm compression or with a penetrating forearm injury should be admitted to the hospital for observation, and if any of the foregoing symptoms or signs develop, the forearm should be decompressed without delay. Occasionally it may be permissible to send a patient home if he or she has a full understanding of what signs to watch for and knows to return at once if any develop.

A compartment syndrome in the upper extremity may also follow heavy prolonged and unaccustomed use of a muscle or group of muscles.[2] The symptom of severe pain and the sign of tense, hard swelling are similar no matter what the cause. Treatment is also the same: release of the constricted muscle.

IATROGENIC DISASTERS

Especially in these days of litigious patients and attorneys willing and eager to press suit, it is important to admit that iatrogenic problems can happen and then take all measures to avoid their occurrence. High-pressure injection injuries and compartment syndrome might be termed potential iatrogenic disasters caused by a physician's lack of knowledge or, put another way, "sins of omission."

Arterial cannulation for diagnostic studies or hemodynamic monitoring of critically ill patients is common practice today. Although patients with indwelling catheters are unlikely to be seen by primary care physicians, patients who have had angiographic studies may well appear in an emergency department when complications develop. With brachial artery cannulation, extravasation of blood may lead to nerve compression within the brachial sheath.[3] If decompression is done as an urgent procedure, long-term nerve impairment is minimal or absent. Radial artery cannulation done carefully is associated with minimal morbidity.[4]

Other sins of omission that are more obvious and less forgiveable include failure to remove constrictive jewelry or clothing; failure to use all diagnostic measures available (especially careful examination and x-ray); failure to give tetanus toxoid or tetanus immune globulin (Hyper-Tet); failure to dress the hand adequately and to make sure that it is kept elevated; and failure to provide access to follow-up.

Sins of commission include overzealous exploration of bloody wounds, with nerve damage inflicted by ill-placed clamps; too lengthy a search for a foreign body may result in the same type of iatrogenic injury. Incautious statements about the absence of any serious injury when in fact there is major nerve or tendon injury may be even more troublesome than the injury itself.

We can only be conscientious and careful with patients and frank in discussing and explaining the actual and potential problems. Certainly no more can be required but we owe the patient at least that much.

PATIENT-CAUSED DISASTERS

Some persons do not cooperate and follow instructions no matter how explicit. Fortunately these people are fairly uncommon.

The one group of patients who inflict tremendous damage upon their bodies in general and their hands in particular are drug addicts. This unfortunate group of unhappy people appear all too often in emergency departments with advanced infections and other hand injuries. Usually venous and lymphatic drainage is already marginal following months or years of destruction by injections. This, of course, compounds the problems of swelling and stiffness that attend any injury.

Often a hand injury has been long neglected in this group of persons, so the chance that infection exists when they are first seen is high. The administration of intravenous antibiotics is often impossible. Finally, drug addicts usually have poor personal hygiene and poor nutrition, both factors compounding the chances of infection and the rapidity of recovery from any injury. These people have to be handled more aggressively in terms of hospital admission for careful scrutiny to avoid major crippling of the upper extremity.

REFERENCES

1. Newmeyer, W. L., and Kilgore, E. S.: Volkmann's ischemic contracture due to soft tissue injury alone. J. Hand Surg. *1*:221–227, 1976.

2. Tompkins, D. G.: Exercise myopathy of the extensor carpi ulnaris muscle. J. Bone Joint Surg., *59A*:407–408, 1977.

3. Braun, R. M.: Injury to the brachial plexus as a result of diagnostic arteriography. Presented at the American Society for Surgery of the Hand, Annual Meeting, Las Vegas, Nevada, February, 1977.

4. Mandel, M. A., and Dauchot, P. J.: Radial artery cannulation in 1,000 patients: precautions and complications. J. Hand Surg., *2*:482–485, 1977.

Amputations

U PPER extremity amputations vary in magnitude from trivial to tremendous. Amputations of the fingerpad lie at the lesser end of the severity scale and have been discussed in Chapter 7 on fingertip injuries. At the other end of the scale are total amputations of whole sections of the upper extremity; it may be possible to reattach these amputations successfully. Between these two extremes lie the subtotal amputations, distal digit amputations, and nonreplantable mangled amputations.

Although amputations account for only about 2% of all hand injuries, there is a great interest in them today because of their replant potential. Patients with amputations who are seen initially in large metropolitan centers are usually referred to specialists with dispatch, but in remote areas with less access to hand surgeons, the primary care physician can render much help in the office or emergency room, and may be the key person in preventing protracted disability. Amputations present the physician with some of the more challenging problems in hand surgery.

Replantation of Amputated Parts

This is one of the frontiers of hand surgery in the mid-1970s.[1] The advent of microsuture material, microsurgical instruments, good microscopes, and surgeons who know how to use them has resulted in some extraordinary achievements. The first physician to see the patient initiates the chain of events that leads to the attempt to replant the part, or conversely, to discard the amputated part.

The technical potential for replanting amputated parts is much

217

greater than the desirability for replanting them. Newspaper stories that trumpet the early successes of replanted parts are rarely followed up in print with the tales of protracted disability, the often multiple procedures that must be done, and the attendant expense and discomfort on the part of the patient. Two questions should be asked when a patient arrives with an amputated part: (1) Can it be replanted? (2) Should it be replanted?

In the hands of skilled microsurgeons, amputations that have occurred near or at the distal joint of a digit are potentially replantable. The sharper the laceration of amputation, the more technically feasible is the replant. However, even with considerable vessel disruption at the two amputation borders, the reestablishment of arterial inflow and venous outflow by the use of autogenous vein grafts may be possible. Digits, hands, or arms that are badly mangled are generally not potentially replantable, especially if the entire amputated part has been torn and shredded or if the remaining stump has suffered extensive damage. On the basis of the wound alone, many amputations are obviously either replantable or not, but there still exist many situations in which the decision is difficult to make (Fig. 13-1).

The second question is more difficult to answer. The decision must be based partly on the physical situation, but to a large extent on the patient's age, occupation, psychologic make-up, and desires.

At the digit level, the thumb is more crucial than any of the other digits. If the thumb is missing at the MCP level, the urgency to replant it is great. The urgency to replant a thumb that has been amputated at the IP level, especially if good flaps remain on the stump (Fig. 13-2), is far less because the thumb is still highly functional. If a single one of the second through fifth digits is gone, the replant urgency drops greatly, although in an individual situation it may be high. For example, a young woman (Fig. 13-3) might suffer more to regain a finger than a laborer who is interested in a pain-free, strong hand. The farther out along the digit the amputation occurs, the less is the urgency to attempt replantation. If multiple digits are amputated, especially at a proximal level, the desirability of attempting to replant at least some of them rises to a higher level.

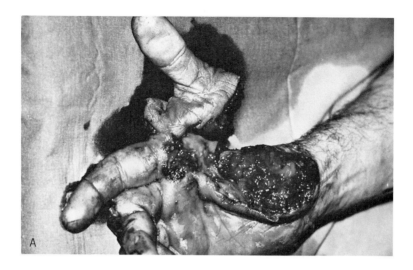

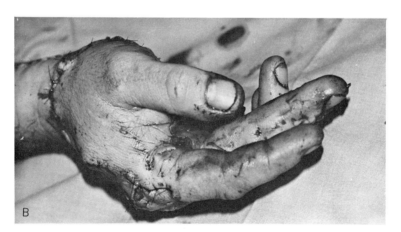

FIG. 13-1.   (A) The right (major) thumb was torn off through the first metacarpal. This is not an ideal situation for replantation. (B) At the conclusion of microsurgical procedures that utilized vein grafts, the thumb is pink and warm.

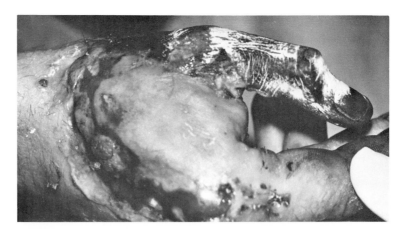

FIG. 13-1.   (C) *The same thumb at 14 days following injury. Failure was probably foreordained because of the ripping, avulsing nature of the injury.*

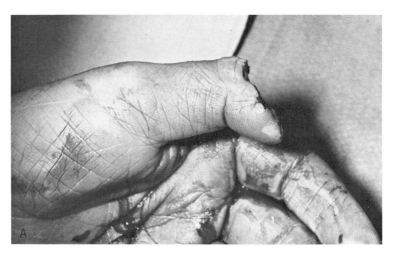

FIG. 13-2.   (A) *A 50-year-old man sawed off this portion of his left (minor) thumb.*

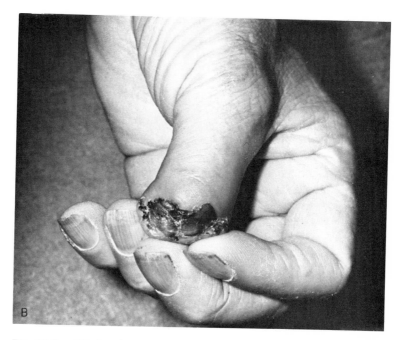

FIG. 13-2. (B) A pain-free, sensible, highly functional thumb resulted following turn-over of the volar flap.

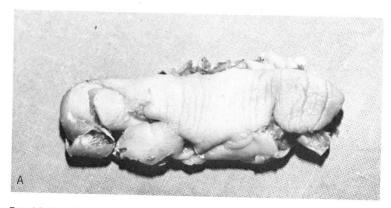

FIG. 13-3. (A) A young woman sustained injuries with a power saw. This is the badly mangled ring finger, which was not considered replantable.

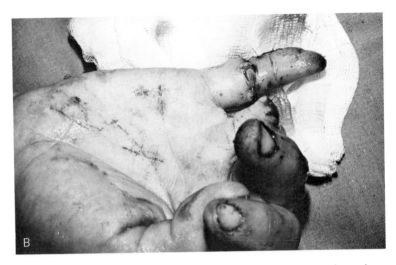

FIG. 13-3. (B) The little finger was successfully replanted, as shown here from the volar aspect.

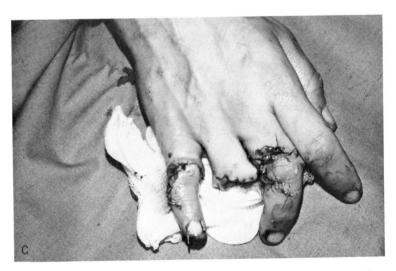

FIG. 13-3. (C) The ring finger stump has enough skin for easy flap closure. The PIP joint of the long finger was destroyed and an immediate silastic joint implant was used to preserve length and function.

It is important to involve the patient and his or her family as much as possible in the decision regarding replantation. The primary care physician should always stress that the attempt to replant will be made if the operating surgeon believes that it is technically possible. After all, the surgeon will be the person doing the work, and should not be forced into an impossible situation by rash promises made at the primary care level (Fig. 13-4)

As the amputation level moves proximally to involve a section of the hand, the entire hand, or more of the extremity, every consideration should be given to attempting replantation. At these levels, the recovery of the functions of sensibility and mobility is more difficult, and the possibility that further operations are needed to attempt restoration of these functions is larger. Always bear in mind that a well-padded, painless stump achieved soon after injury has much to recommend it, especially when compared to a painful replanted part that remains functionless and clinging tenuously to life (Fig. 13-5).

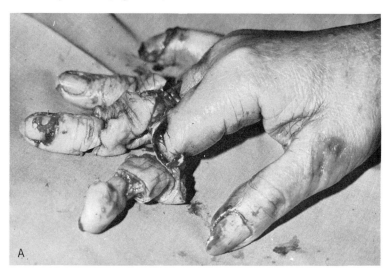

Fig. 13-4. *(A) A middle-aged woman caught these fingers in a meat grinder. General anesthesia was necessary to extricate the extremity. To raise even a glimmer of hope for replantation would be unfortunate and unfair to this patient.*

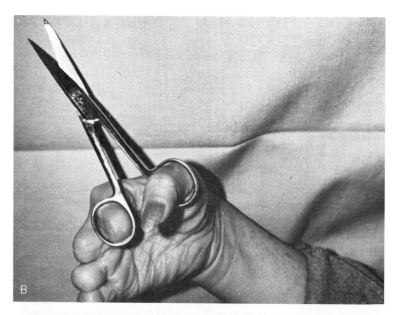

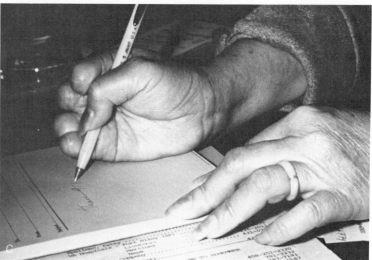

FIG. 13-4. (B,C) Function following injury was good and she had no pain.

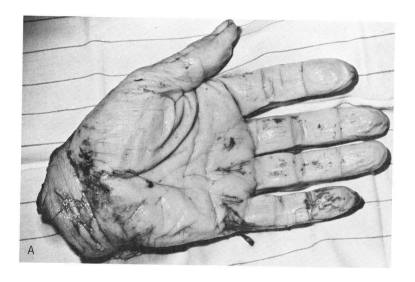

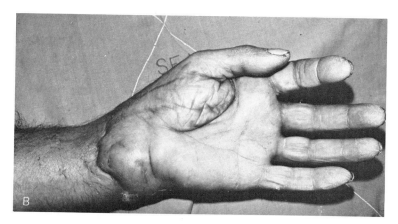

FIG. 13-5. (A) *This self-inflicted amputation was done with a kitchen knife by a greatly disturbed patient. (B) The replanted hand was technically successful. Function was poor and the patient was unable to comprehend what had happened or to participate in rehabilitation.*

PREPARATION FOR REPLANTATION

If the decision has been made to refer the patient for attempted replantation of a limb or digit, no time should be wasted. Digits may be successfully replanted as much as 24 hours after amputation if they have been stored properly, but hands or larger segments of the upper extremity undergo irreversible muscle necrosis much sooner. For these parts, six hours between amputation and restoration of arterial inflow is probably the maximal allowable time.

The amputated part should be placed in a sterile container, or if it is too large, wrapped in sterile towels that are made waterproof with some type of cellophane wrap, such as Saran Wrap or a 3-M towel drape. The entire package is then put into a basin containing ice and water, which will keep it at about 4°C. Irrigation of the vessels is not indicated with amputated digits. With the hand or forearm, flushing may be necessary, but this is best left to the surgical replant team. Manipulation of the vessels is a time-wasting procedure in the emergency department and may actually destroy vessels and make the replantation more difficult technically.

The amputation stump should be treated minimally. Any hemorrhage should be stopped by compression or if necessary, vessel ligation. Nonadherent gauze covered with sponges soaked in povidone iodine makes a good dressing. Cast padding and a light plaster shell or a splint and bias-cut stockinette may be put over the dressing. Support the arm at heart level. If the patient is to be admitted to the same hospital into which he or she has first been brought, start an intravenous infusion using a large needle or catheter and perform the routine admission blood analyses immediately. In many cases it is wise to type and cross-match blood, but in every situation a clot should be saved for this purpose. Administer antibiotics (usually a cephalosporin) intravenously and give either tetanus immune globulin or tetanus toxoid.

If the patient is to be transported to another facility for replantation, the same steps are taken except that the tests done for blood type and cross-match and the routine laboratory studies are performed on arrival at the receiving institution. Often pain is not a problem, but if it is, give analgesics intramuscularly. Although some surgeons prefer to perform replantations using regional block anesthesia, the patient should be put on NPO status as soon as he or she arrives in the emergency department. Depending on the patient's age and medical history, an electrocardiogram and chest roentgenogram may be necessary.

While all these steps are being carried out, the primary care physician should contact the surgeon who is going to attempt the replantation and relay as much information about the patient as possible. This allows the receiving institution (if the patient is to be transported) to be ready to commence surgery soon after the patient's arrival. Haste without oversight in preparation is the crucial first step to successful replantation.

Nonreplantable Amputations

The majority of amputations are not potentially or practically replantable. In many amputations, both the amputated part and the stump have been severely mangled (see Fig. 13-4). Sometimes the amputated part is lost. Often, especially when a single digit is involved, the better part of valor is not to attempt replantation. The single digit that is probably most expendable is the index finger. The long finger readily assumes the role of the index finger in the pinch function. In reality, patients automatically use the long finger in this function if the index finger is painful or short. In the case of a troublesome index stump, the index ray can be removed creating a wider thumb web space and a cosmetically acceptable hand that functions well (Fig. 13-6).

The loss of one of the ulnar three digits leads to a loss of gripping power. If the long finger or ring finger is absent at the MCP level, a troublesome "hole" in the hand causes one to lose small objects grasped in the palm (Fig. 13-7). This situation is best treated by transferring the single adjacent ray to the position of the amputated ray. In the situation shown in Figure 13-7, the index ray was transferred to the long finger ray at the level of the proximal metacarpal. Loss of the little finger reduces the hand breadth, but the ulnar border of the hand may be tailored cosmetically.

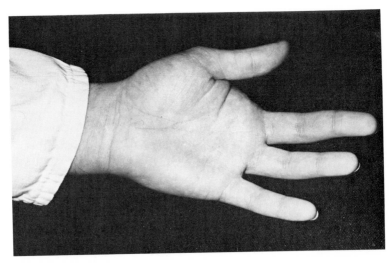

FIG. 13-6.   *This young man had a tender index finger stump that he was constantly bumping. Index ray amputation provided an excellent cosmetic and functional result.*

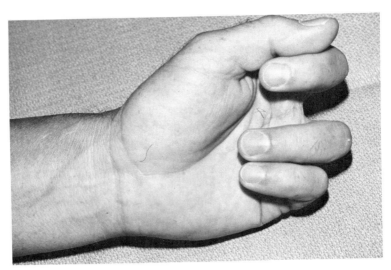

FIG. 13-7.   *This "hole" in the hand can be troublesome because small items drop through the gap.*

Emergency Stump Management

When seen initially, a patient with an amputation deemed not suitable for replantation should be treated with the usual support measures that have been outlined previously. If the patient can be readily referred to a specialist, that is often the wisest course of action. However, much initial surgery can be performed in the emergency department or physician's office. An initial roentgenogram is usually helpful.

Always use anesthesia, a tourniquet, and a sterile field. Avoid blindly clamping vessels. If the vessels are bleeding, they may be clamped discretely when the tourniquet is inflated. Remove loose bits of bone. Snip shreds of tendon. Obviously nonviable skin should be debrided, but leave marginal skin in place. If this marginal skin survives, closure is made easier, and little is lost if it dies.

Never pull tendon ends down and attach them to the bone. Cut free tendon ends and allow them to retract. If they are sutured to bone ends, the entire tendon mechanism may be thrown off balance and adjacent fingers will not work satisfactorily.

Digital nerves often are not easy to identify. They lie, along with digital arteries, in loose volar fat on the ulnar-volar and radial-volar sides of the digit. Nerves are mesenteric structures that will not retract much if they are pulled down and cut off. If they can be identified, free them for about a centimeter and push them back under the skin flaps, so that the neuroma that develops will not be caught in scar tissue (see Chapter 14). In formal operative revisions of amputations, the nerves are actually sutured under skin flaps remote from the wound. By placing the neuroma under dorsal flaps, much trouble with painful tingling at a pressure point may be avoided.

If the amputation is through a joint, or so close to a joint that removal of bone fragments exposes an articular surface, the articular surface does not need to be removed. If necessary, the condylar flares may be nipped with a rongeur to permit skin closure, but there is no reason per se to remove the cartilaginous surface of the bone.

The key to successful amputation closure is adequate amounts of skin; tight closure invariably leads to problems of pain and tenderness. The skin flaps that can be developed should lie loosely over the amputation stump. It is better to shorten a digit and achieve a loose closure than attempt to save more of a digit and have a tight closure. The exact fashion in which the flaps are brought over a stump depends on the nature of the amputation. If a flap can be brought either across the end of the stump or alternatively over a central portion of it, bring it across the end and leave a gap in the middle portion to heal by granulation or by a split-thickness skin graft (Fig. 13-8). The ideal situation is one in which the amputation inclines obliquely from dorsal-proximal to volar-distal, because a volar flap can be turned up to provide excellent cover of the stump. The flaps often do not come together perfectly and a so-called dog-ear may occur at one or more corners; in general, do not spend a great amount of time fussing with these. If the flaps have a good blood supply and no postinjury swelling or infection has occurred, healing and molding take place.

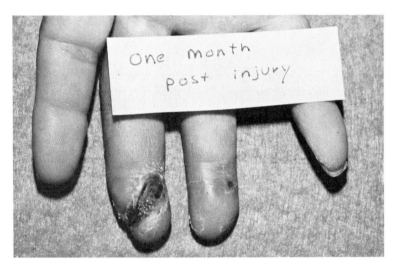

FIG. 13-8. *A flap was used to cover the distal finger. Ordinarily the gap would be filled in with a split-thickness skin graft, but the patient decided nature would do the job fast enough.*

The same principles of primary care apply to more proximal amputations as apply to digital amputations. However, patients with more proximal amputations usually need to be referred for operative revision and closure because of the size and number of structures involved. Primary care principles are to stop hemorrhage and suture the skin edges without tension. Apply an appropriate dressing and institute other support measures as discussed previously.

Even if a digit or part of a digit is apparently hopelessly mangled, saving viable parts of it may aid in later reconstructive procedures. For example, if the entire dorsal surface of a finger including bones and joints has been injured irreparably but the volar skin remains in viable condition, it should be saved. In some instances this retained flap can be used to resurface other areas (Fig. 13-9).

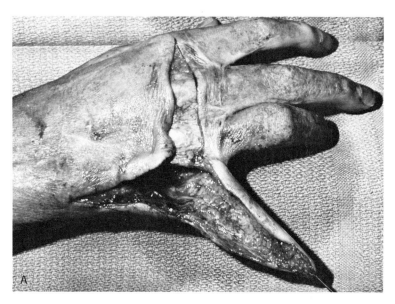

Fig. 13-9.   (A) *This young man had a burn that resulted in tight dorsal skin and a fifth digit that was functionless but had good volar skin. The skeletal structures were filleted out of the fifth digit and the dorsal skin was released.*

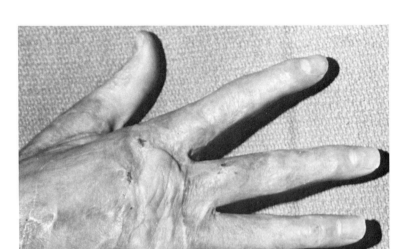

FIG. 13-9.   (B) *Some months later, the volar skin flap from the little finger has healed well, permitting much more mobility in the remaining digits.*

As in all aspects of hand injury, the course of action to be taken is that which maximizes recovery and minimizes disability time. Even with extensive loss a determined patient can make a remarkable functional recovery (see Fig. 13-4).

REFERENCES

1. Weiland, A. J., et al.: Replantation of digits and hands: Analysis of surgical techniques and functional results in 71 patients with 86 replantations. J. Hand Surg., 2:1–12, 1977.

14

Nerve Injuries

THE main role of the primary care physician in the treatment of nerve injuries is accurate diagnosis. However, in certain closed injuries and various entrapment problems, a more active role may be played by the judicious injection of combinations of cortisone and lidocaine and by appropriate splinting.

Examination for Nerve Injuries

With any nerve lesion, there is partial or complete loss of sensibility or muscle function or both. The key to accurate diagnosis is to find an area of function as isolated as possible and concentrate testing on that particular area.

LOSS OF SENSIBILITY

The nerves responsible for sensibility overlap variously on the pads of the digits and the dorsum of the hand (see pp. 14, 17). On the digits especially, certain objective signs are useful for detecting loss of sensibility. The sympathetic fibers travel with the major nerve trunks. When a sensory or mixed nerve is lost, the area that it serves will be anhidrotic. This is a striking finding in late nerve lesions, and it may also be present in the acute situation. This sign is especially useful for patients who are unable to cooperate well, such as children. If the patient is not sweating, a corollary of this test is the skin-wrinkling assessment. Ordinarily, the fingerpads become wrinkled when immersed in warm water for a few minutes, but denervated fingerpads will not wrinkle upon immersion. This may be a useful test on occasions.

The more time-honored methods of testing sensibility should not be overlooked. When testing for sensation, it is important that the patient not be distracted. This means that he or she should be comfortably recumbent and as pain-free as possible without the use of a local or regional anesthetic or heavy doses of analgesics. It is unlikely that much useful information can be gained about the status of sensibility by active testing in patients who are hysterical or intoxicated, or with whom the examiner does not share a common language, or who are too young to understand.

The two objects useful for testing sensibility are a cotton-tipped applicator with a piece of the cotton drawn out and a sharp object, such as a no. 25 needle. First establish "normal" feeling reactions with the patient by testing a clearly uninjured area with a similar sensory supply. The normal and suspected pathologic areas are then tested alternately applying the same amount of force, which should not be great. The most information will be gained on the first "pass." Persistence in testing fatigues and confuses the patient. Occasionally it may be wise to let the patient rest for a few minutes and then return for another session.

If the direct test for sensibility does not help and the signs of loss of sensibility are equivocal, you have to rely on the location and depth of the wound as the best indicator of nerve injury. Certain wounding agents are notorious for their deep penetration and subsequent nerve injury. These include lacerations with all types of glass and similar materials such as ceramics.

If numbness accompanies a wound that is more crushing in nature, the chances are that only a severe contusion, known as a neurapraxia, has occurred; full recovery is most likely. A nerve that is functionally interrupted but anatomically intact, as may occur with a severe stretch injury, is said to have axonotmesis. Total anatomic severance is called neurotmesis. Neurapraxia and neurotmesis are the most frequently encountered clinical conditions. Axonotmesis may be seen in severe traction injuries, such as brachial plexus stretch injuries; otherwise it is uncommon in the hand and forearm.

If you cannot definitively ascertain the status of sensibility, carefully explain the situation to the patient in terminology that he or she can comprehend, and give extra impetus to the need for follow-up.

When a definite diagnosis of a divided sensory nerve is made near the time of injury, refer the patient immediately to a hand surgeon. The timing of repair will vary with the individual surgeon, but in the case of multiple nerve injury especially, early repair (within a day or two of injury) may be preferred. Fortunately, little is lost if the repair is delayed slightly beyond that time.

Two long-term problems appear when sensory nerves are not repaired. The first, obviously, is lack of sensibility of the affected part. However, the problem that more often troubles the patient, especially if the involved area is not critical for sensibility, is a sensitive neuroma. A neuroma is the formation of a mass of jumbled axons by the proximal stump of the nerve in an effort to regenerate itself. Particularly if a neuroma becomes trapped in scar tissue, it is hypersensitive to the lightest touch, such as a sleeve going across it, the pressure of a watch band or ring, or even light gripping or grasping. Once a neuroma pattern has been well established it may be impossible to break. If a neuroma is attacked early, either by repair of the nerve or by transfer to a protected area free of scar (for example, under a muscle belly), the problem usually vanishes. This is the reason why nerves should not be left near amputation stumps, but should be dissected free and deliberately placed elsewhere in a protected area.

Patients often ask the primary care physician about the chances for recovery from a nerve injury and the rate of recovery. Nerves regenerate at a rate of 1 mm. per day, and this regeneration probably begins several days after injury. The rate of functional recovery is much slower than the rate of actual nerve progression. In a purely sensory nerve the chances of functional recovery after an adequate repair are high, possibly up to 80 to 90 percent. This recovery may not be complete for many months. Even three or four years after injury patients still note increasing levels of sensibility.

Assessment of recovery is made by the various signs and tests of sensibility. The presence of Tinel's sign in an area of previously lost sensibility is firm evidence of recovery. This is elicited by tapping in the area of the lost sensibility and having the patient note an electric-shock feeling. Remember, however, that tapping the area of injury or repair is an indication, if Tinel's sign is present, of no purposeful regeneration. When Tinel's sign disappears from the area of injury-repair and appears when the numb area is tapped, nerve recovery is taking place. For a time after nerve repair, tingling will occur at the site of injury-repair and in the area of lost sensibility distal to the injury. In the case of large nerves, Tinel's sign at the repair site or graft site may never entirely disappear.

Patients may ask about the restoration of sensibility to areas where critical sensible tissue has been hopelessly lost; this is especially true of the thumb pad. If the rest of the hand is relatively spared from injury, a thumb pad may be resurfaced with a neurovascular-island pedicle flap, formed from one-half of the pad of another finger on its own neurovascular stalk. Usually this flap is taken from the ulnar side of the ring finger, because the operation was first used in total median nerve loss and this was the closest sensible pad to the thumb. The defect on the donor finger is covered with split-thickness skin graft and sensibility is sacrificed in that area. Sensibility in the transferred flap may be good, but rarely is it normal. The patient usually makes at least a functional cortical transfer so that the pad will be a "thumb" pad, instead of a long finger or ring fingerpad. The ability to discern two points close together, which in the normal finger is 4 to 6 mm., rarely gets below 7 to 9 mm. in a neurovascular island pedicle.

LOSS OF MOTOR POWER

The other critical function of nerves is to carry the impulse to activate various muscles. In the hand, 15 intrinsic muscles are innervated by the ulnar nerve and 5 are innervated by the median nerve. Of the 24 extrinsic muscles, the median nerve innervates 9; the ulnar nerve, 3; and the radial nerve, 12.

Testing for motor loss demands a sound appreciation of functional anatomy. Although some repetition of anatomy follows here, a review of Chapter 1 may be in order.

In assessing motor loss, the examiner must form an hypothesis regarding laceration injury to motor nerves and then confirm or deny the theory by testing with as much precision as possible. This means finding an easily isolated motor unit with little variable or cross-innervation.

Certain nerves are easier to test than others, and the ease of testing may depend on the level of the laceration. Localizing the acute condition as closely as possible is useful for subsequent treating physicians. In the acute state, a nerve may function that subsequently becomes neurapraxic due to edema. Knowing that it was functioning initially and is therefore intact is highly useful.

Specific Nerve Lesions

These lesions are discussed in the order of proximal to distal. Three major mixed nerves—the radial, the ulnar, and the median—are considered, as well as the terminal sensory branches of the median and the ulnar nerves, or the so-called digital nerves.

RADIAL NERVE

Fractures, lacerations, and prolonged compression are the most common causes of injuries to this nerve. In the case of a humeral fracture, it is vulnerable to injury at the point where the nerve circles behind the humerus. The nerve may be lacerated entirely, severely contused, or even trapped in the fracture line. Whenever a midshaft humeral fracture is seen, radial nerve function should be tested by asking the patient to extend his wrist, thumb, and then the other digits. The presence or absence of radial nerve function should be noted.

Penetrating injuries may result in partial or total division of the radial nerve at any level of its course, but most commonly this occurs along the outer, lower one-third of the humerus and in the muscle mass distal to the lateral epicondyle. The muscles are innervated in sequence, and a careful examination may locate the lesion precisely.

The main trunk of the radial nerve gives off motor branches to the brachioradialis (BR) and extensor carpi radialis longus (ECRL) muscles before dividing into the superficial radial sensory nerve and the posterior interosseus nerve. The latter innervates, in order, the extensor carpi radialis brevis (ECRB), the supinator, the extensor digitorum communis (EDC), the extensor digiti minimi (EDM), the extensor pollicis longus (EPL), the extensor pollicis brevis (EPB), the abductor pollicis longus (APL), and the extensor indicis proprius (EIP). In the case of a penetrating injury that results in a loss of digit extension but with wrist extension maintained, the lesion can be localized. This may greatly aid future management, because it places the injury at a level where the nerve has arborized, and injuries at this level are much harder to repair than main trunk injuries.

Penetrating injuries may be either clean-cut and exact, as occurs with a knife or piece of glass, or they may be diffuse, as from a gunshot wound. With the latter, a profound neurapraxia may last for several months but function ultimately recovers fully. If nerve function is gone after a sharp wound, there will probably be no recovery, and earlier consideration should be given to referral for tendon transfer or secondary nerve repair by an appropriate method.

To test for radial nerve motor function, brace the forearm on the table or other platform with the wrist and digits hanging free. Then ask the patient to extend first the wrist, then the thumb, and finally the other digits. An estimate of the alacrity and force of extension may be made (Figs. 14-1 and 14-2). Differentiation of specific extensors may be made according to the sequence discussed previously. Remember that digital interphalangeal extension will occur and be forceful even with complete radial palsy. The exception is that thumb IP extension will be weak, and hyperextension at this joint will not occur.

The consequence of injury to the superficial sensory branch of the radial nerve does not lie so much in the loss of sensibility as it does in the development of a supersensitive neuroma. The autogenous area of sensibility of this nerve is the dorsal thumb web. The nerve is especially prone to injury on the radial, dorsal, distal forearm. At this level it emerges from beneath the protecting brachioradialis and lies very close to the skin. An apparently innocuous laceration may injure it and begin a vicious cycle of

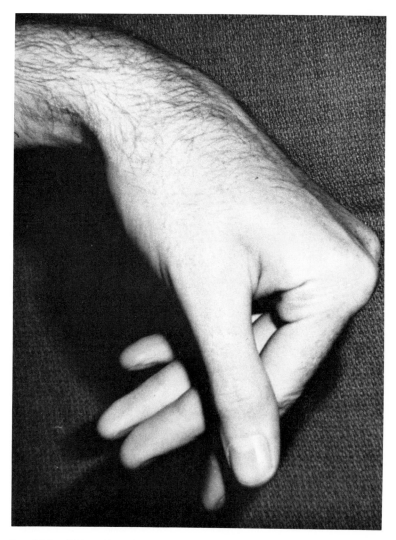

FIG. 14-1. *This patient has complete radial nerve palsy due to laceration of the nerve. There is no wrist or MCP extension; weak thumb IP extension is possible owing to intact intrinsics.*

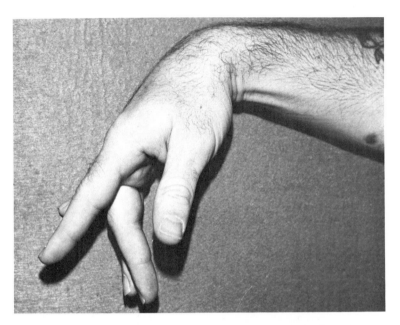

FIG. 14-2.   *Incomplete radial nerve palsy due to the blast effect of a gun shot wound. Over a period of six months, recovery was almost complete.*

neuroma pain that is difficult to eradicate. For this reason early diagnosis and referral of patients with this lesion is desirable.

MEDIAN NERVE

The median nerve injury most commonly seen by the primary care physician is a partial or total laceration at the wrist. The median nerve traverses the forearm deep to the sublimis muscle bellies until just before reaching the wrist. At wrist level it emerges to lie just under the skin, antebrachial fascia, and palmaris longus if present. The nerve then dips beneath the thick volar carpal ligament, where it is once again well protected. It should be assumed that any laceration across the low volar forearm and wrist harbors an injured median nerve (Fig. 14-3). Knives, razor

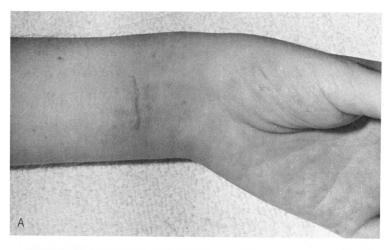

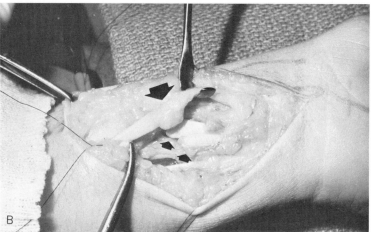

FIG. 14-3. (A) *This young woman complained of spotty numbness in the median nerve distribution and difficulty with index and long finger flexion. Two or three months previously she had lacerated her forearm with glass while intoxicated and had gone to a local emergency department, where the wound was sutured after a cursory examination. (B) Operative exposure revealed a large neuroma at the site of the median nerve laceration (large arrow) and two divided flexor tendons (small arrows). Always suspect deep injury with glass lacerations.*

blades, and broken glass are the most common injuring agents. Glass is a particularly insidious agent because shards can penetrate deeply, sometimes leaving superficial structures intact. A knife or razor blade is more likely to cut everything in its path.

If the wound is self-inflicted, the patient is usually hysterical and uncooperative. Even if the injury was purely accidental, the patient may be so upset that an accurate examination is difficult. Be wary of drawing definitive conclusions regarding the status of the nerve on the basis of thumb pronation and opposition. Frequently the ulnar-innervated flexor pollicis brevis overlaps sufficiently to allow what appears to be very good thumb pronation and opposition. Full thumb pronation and opposition requires that the nails of the thumb and opposed finger lie 180 degrees from each other (Fig. 14-4).

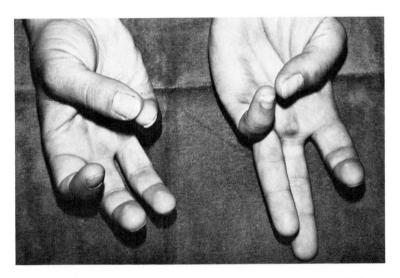

FIG. 14-4. *This young man has median nerve palsy of the left hand (right of photograph) due to a wrist laceration that severed the median nerve. The right thumb and little finger can be brought pad to pad with the nails 180 degrees from each other. The left thumb pad can only be brought to the side of the little finger with the nails about 90 degrees apart. This is a subtle test and difficult to interpret accurately with an acute injury.*

Sensibility in the median nerve distribution is a more reliable test of function. The autonomous areas should be carefully tested and compared with normal areas of similar critical levels of sensibility. In practice, this means comparing the pads of the index finger, thumb, or long finger with the little fingerpad. Remember that a partial laceration may produce an apparently bizarre sensory pattern. Be wary about assuring the patient that no injury exists. Little is lost if the nerve is not repaired immediately, but a patient may become hostile and upset if he or she has been blithely assured that there was no nerve injury and then experiences significant nerve loss.

The median nerve is injured less frequently at other levels of the forearm, and then only with deeply penetrating lacerations. It is possible to have a narrow laceration that damages the nerve, but usually the wound is a wide gaping one, and the nerve injury is only part of the problem.

The median nerve is infrequently injured distal to the wrist because of the protection of skin, palmar fascia, and volar carpal ligament. However, occasionally penetrating trauma that appears trivial at first glance may injure the nerve. When porcelain handles on faucets were common, they caused a typical injury. As the patient forcefully pushed the handle, it would break and the penetrating porcelain shards would injure the nerve. This particular area is difficult for the hand surgeon to repair because the nerve arborizes into the digital nerves and lies just under the superficial transverse vascular arch.

ULNAR NERVE

This nerve is injured less commonly than the median nerve. Except at the elbow, where it lies just under the skin and fascia in the groove of the medial epicondyle, it is well protected. However, the most common site of laceration is at the wrist, which often occurs in conjunction with median nerve laceration. The ulnar artery is usually lacerated when the nerve is cut.

Loss of the ulnar nerve at wrist level or above means loss of the ulnar-innervated hand intrinsic muscles. The most specific test for function is the contraction of the first dorsal interosseus muscle, which is obvious when the patient places his hand on its ulnar side and elevates the index finger (please refer to Fig. 1-12).

A crude but more rapid test is abduction-adduction of the second through fifth digits, which is more reliable than the motor test for the median nerve. A patient with an ulnar nerve motor loss loses good pinch. The thumb goes into IP flexion because loss of the adductor pollicis forces the flexor pollicis longus to provide most of the power. This is called Froment's sign (Fig. 14-5A).

Clawing of the ring and little fingers is the other characteristic hand stance with an ulnar palsy. All interossei and the lumbrical muscles to the ring finger and the little finger are paralyzed, with resultant unopposed or unbalanced force from the extrinsic muscles. This causes the typical "intrinsic minus" hand, with MCP hyperextension and IP furling (Fig. 14-5B).

Ulnar nerve sensibility is confined to the ulnar side of the hand, the little finger, and the ulnar half of the ring finger. The volar branches of the nerve cover the fingerpads and eponychial area. The remainder of the dorsal fingers and hand are given sensibility by the dorsal sensory branch of the nerve, which arises above the wrist.

DIGITAL NERVES

Although these purely sensory nerves are branches of the ulnar and the median nerves, they deserve separate consideration as entities in themselves. Once they have branched off the parent nerves, they lie fairly superficially and are prone to laceration and compressive trauma.

The two nerves to the thumb lie on the fascia of the thumb intrinsic muscles, and they pass into the digit close to the flexor tendon sheath and close to one another. These two nerves and the border nerves to the index finger and the little finger are the most critical sensory nerves in the hand. The border nerves are proper nerves from the point of their origin in contrast to the other six nerves, which arise as common sensory nerves and then split to become proper nerves.

The radial digital nerve to the index finger and the ulnar digital nerve to the little finger lie superficially on the volar borders of the

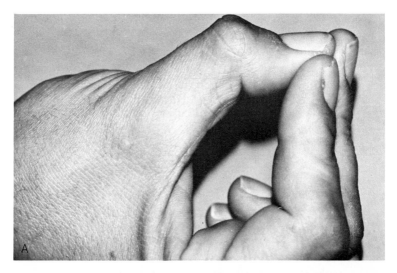

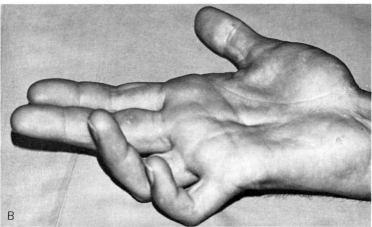

FIG. 14-5. (A) This patient is a young man with an ulnar motor palsy due to laceration of the nerve at wrist level. The thumb flexing at the IP joint in pinch is called Froment's sign; it is characteristic of the lesion because the flexor pollicis longus tries to compensate for the lost adductor pollicis. (B) Clawing of the ring and little fingers in the same patient. Only the little lumbrical muscles prevent this deformity from occurring in the long and index fingers as well.

radial and ulnar sides of the hand. Isolated injuries in these areas often result in injury to these nerves. The early repair of these four nerves (i.e., the two to the thumb and the index and the little finger border nerves), is more important than the repair of the other six.

The other six digital nerves arise from their parent nerves as common sensory nerves, splitting to become proper sensory nerves and giving sensibility to the adjacent sides of the second through the fifth digits. The nerves traverse the palm deep to the accompanying digital artery, but come to lie superficial to the artery as they enter the digit. This, of course, is the reason why spurting blood from a digital wound is good evidence that a digital nerve has been lacerated (Fig. 14-6).

Digital nerves are reparable at least to the DIP joint level. Beyond this point the arborization results in fine filaments that might be repaired microsurgically, but the results do not always justify the effort required.

All digital nerve injuries should be diagnosed as accurately as possible, and, if injury is suspected, the patient should be referred expeditiously, if not urgently, to a hand surgeon for repair. Injuries to a thumb nerve, border nerve, or both nerves in a single digit pose somewhat more urgent situations than an isolated single nerve injury in the central digit. However, remember that any nerve that is not repaired has the potential to become a painful neuroma.

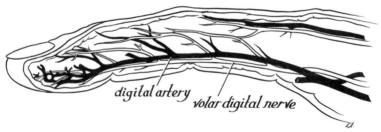

FIG. 14-6.   *The anatomic relationship of the digital artery and nerve changes as the two enter the digit. Note that in the digit the artery lies dorsal to the nerve.*

Nerve Compression or Entrapment Syndromes

Each of the three major nerves to the hand is subject to one or more compression neuropathies. These injuries are generally neurapraxias that may progress to axonotmesis, although this is rare. The terminal motor and sensory branches of the median and ulnar nerves are prone to the same compression problems. The neuropathy may be caused by either a squeezing phenomenon within an anatomic canal or result from prolonged external compression of a nerve against the bone. A combination of these two situations may also occur.

RADIAL NERVE

The classic radial nerve palsy is the so-called Saturday Night Palsy. The patient is unable to extend the wrist, the thumb at the MCP and IP joints, and the other digits at the MCP joints. He or she may also have some numbness over the dorsal-radial low forearm and hand. The most typical history given is that the patient became inebriated and lapsed into unconsciousness with his or her arm draped over a table or chair, compressing the posterior midhumerus. Of course, this is the spot at which the radial nerve encircles the shaft of the humerus. The palsy may vary in both the extent of the involvement and the degree of motor loss.

This injury does not happen only to the "down and out" members of society, and it may follow the use of intoxicants and depressants other than alcohol. The common denominator of injury is prolonged compression at the midhumeral level. A person in an ordinary sleep state would awaken enough to turn and take pressure off the nerve.

The immediate and in most cases definitive treatment is giving reassurance that the defect will correct itself with time. The patient should be provided with a custom-made wrist splint to hold the wrist in about 10 to 15 degrees of extension, since this puts the hand into a position where it can function adequately. Most definitely follow the patient until full recovery has taken place. If recovery is prolonged, electrical conduction studies of the nerve and electromyographic studies of the involved muscles should be obtained. These can be repeated to follow progression. In a rare instance the nerve does not recover and tendon transfers are necessary to correct the deficits.

Other radial nerve compression neuropathies are possible but not common. A primary care physician might encounter radial sensory neurapraxia at the low forearm level. A brisk blow to the nerve in this area may produce transient paresthesia, but persistence of this is most uncommon.

MEDIAN NERVE

The quintessential neuropathy is that of the median nerve at the wrist, or the so-called carpal tunnel syndrome. The median nerve enters the hand in the carpal tunnel in the company of the nine flexor tendons. This canal is 3 to 4 cm. long, and the walls are absolutely unyielding. Tendons are surrounded by synovium, which has the potential for accumulating fluid with swelling. If this should occur, the median nerve is the first structure to suffer. The patient notices numbness and tingling in the sensory distribution of the nerve, which innervates the pads of the thumb, the index finger, the long finger, and the radial side of the ring finger. Sometimes only part of the nerve distribution is affected. Invariably, the symptoms are worse at night and often accompanied by pain, probably because at night the hand assumes the position of rest-injury or wrist flexion. This position aggravates the problem, and it is the basis of the well-known Phalen test. In this test the examiner holds the wrist in flexion. If paresthesias are produced within a minute or so, the test is considered positive. Unless the patient is unusually astute, he or she complains that the entire hand becomes numb and often attributes this to poor circulation. Patients often recount awakening at night to shake the hand to "wake it up."

The onset of the carpal tunnel syndrome is usually insidious and without an obvious cause. However, recognized physiologic states may cause the syndrome. Any fluid retention state may cause carpal tunnel syndrome symptoms. It is commonly seen in pregnant women, and it may be worse in women in the premenstrual phase of their ovulatory cycle. A diuretic often provides relief to this group of patients.

Specific trauma may cause a carpal tunnel syndrome. The problem is often seen after a Colles' fracture and surgical release may be necessary. It occurs in working persons who use their hands as a hammer (such as sheet-metal workers who bang conduits into place), and in those whose hands are submitted to repetitive trauma (jackhammer operators). I have seen two patients, both doctors who bicycle for pleasure, who have intermittent symptoms caused by gripping the handlebars. When a specific cause can be identified, a change in the pattern of using the hands is necessary. If the symptoms persist after this change, surgery may be necessary, but surgery without a change in the causative factor is worthless.

The disease most commonly associated with carpal tunnel syndrome is rheumatoid arthritis. In this case the cause of the syndrome is proliferation of the synovium and surgery is often necessary both to relieve pressure on the nerve and to prevent tendon rupture.

Most patients with carpal tunnel symptoms are seen long before the advanced stage of the disease develops, which is marked by unremitting pain and numbness accompanied by wasting of the thenar musculature on the radial side of the long thumb flexor. When a patient is seen with the problem this advanced, the diagnosis is obvious and immediate referral for early surgery is indicated.

In the more usual, less advanced case, the diagnosis is made by the history and a few simple physical findings. The patient may have a positive Tinel's sign (electric-shock-like tingling) when the nerve is tapped at the wrist level. The Phalen's test described previously is usually positive. There may be some slight thenar atrophy and weakness of thumb opposition-pronation (see Fig. 14-4). The involved fingerpads may have diminished two-point discrimination and loss of sweat.

Relief is often provided by fashioning a cock-up splint to hold the wrist in 10 to 15 degrees of extension; this is worn at night. In addition, one may inject a combination of one of the cortisone drugs, such as triamcinolone (Kenalog), and a local anesthetic into the carpal tunnel. A useful combination is 1 ml. of Kenalog-40 and 2 ml. of 1% plain lidocaine (Xylocaine). The injection technique is the same as that described for median nerve block pp. 69–70). These two measures—the injection and the splint—are both diagnostic and therapeutic. If they do not help to relieve the symptoms, you may order electrical conduction studies of the nerve and electromyographic studies of muscle. At this point the patient should probably be referred to a hand surgeon.

The median nerve is also subject to compression neuropathy in the upper forearm at the point where it passes between the heads of the pronator teres muscle. Symptoms are much the same as with the carpal tunnel syndrome, but in addition, the patient has some loss of flexion of the thumb IP joint and both IP joints of the index finger. Tinel's sign may be positive in the midforearm; Phalen's test will be negative. This compression neuropathy usually requires surgical release and early referral to a surgeon is in order.

ULNAR NERVES

The ulnar nerve is liable to compression at both the elbow and wrist levels. At the elbow level, the nerve passes beneath the medial epicondyle in the so-called cubital tunnel. It may be compressed at this point or just distally, where it passes through the two heads of the flexor carpi ulnaris. Repetitive trauma from leaning on the elbow or banging with the elbow may cause symptoms of paresthesia in the ulnar nerve sensory distribution and ultimately cause weakness in the flexor carpi ulnaris, the two ulnar profundi, and the ulnar-innervated intrinsic muscles. When people speak of hitting their "funny bone," they actually have hit the ulnar nerve at this level.

Although some physicians occasionally inject local anesthetics in the cubital tunnel to induce an ulnar nerve block, this practice should be discouraged because it may lead to symptoms of ulnar neuropathy. This tunnel is tight and contains only the nerve. I have seen some instances of probable iatrogenic neuropathy, and injection at this location seems imprudent.

The ulnar nerve passes from the elbow to the wrist level unencumbered by potential obstacles. It enters the hand through Guyon's canal. This canal contains only the ulnar nerve and artery, and hence it is not subject to the vagaries of synovial swelling. Uncommonly the canal may be tight and give rise to volar sensory loss in the little finger and the ulnar side of the ring finger, as well as causing weakness or even complete motor loss in the ulnar-innervated intrinsic muscle. Just distal to the canal, the intrinsic muscle motor nerve curves around the hook of the hamate bone, where it may be injured by compression against this bony prominence. Fractures of the hook of the hamate may cause motor neuropathy, but fracture is not necessary for the symptoms to appear. If this motor nerve is compressed either acutely or chronically without accompanying sensory loss to give an early warning of the disorder, the patient may find it a rather frightening and mysterious experience. Indeed, the first symptom that the patient may notice is notable clumsiness due to intrinsic muscle paralysis. The diagnosis is made on the basis of the history and a careful examination.

With compression neuropathy of the ulnar nerve at the elbow level, one would expect to find a positive Tinel's sign at the cubital tunnel or just distally, some motor loss of both ulnar-innervated extrinsic and intrinsic muscles, and some dorsal and volar sensory loss in the ulnar side of the hand. With a compression lesion at the level of Guyon's canal level or distally, you would expect to see an alteration or loss of volar sensibility on the little finger and the ulnar side of the ring finger, some motor loss of ulnar-innervated intrinsic muscles, but no dorsal sensory loss and no extrinsic muscle motor loss.

Treatment of ulnar nerve compression neuropathies in the primary care setting consists of the application of a foam rubber elbow pad if the problem occurs at the elbow level, or a splint similar to that used for a median carpal tunnel syndrome if the problem exists at the wrist level. If early relief is not forthcoming with these measures, the patient should be referred promptly to a hand surgeon.

DIGITAL NERVES

Any one of these nerves may undergo neurapraxia from either repetitive trauma or compression from a single blow. Possibly the best known single entity is the so-called bowler's thumb, in which a neuroma incontinuity develops in one of the thumb digital nerves owing to the manner in which the ball is grasped. In this and similar neurapraxias of digital nerves, the treatment is avoidance of the specific causative trauma. Recovery usually occurs over time.

NECK COMPRESSION SYNDROMES

Occasionally one may encounter patients who complain of a numbness in the hand that does not seem to fit any specific nerve disorder despite careful examination and questioning. In such a situation you should suspect a thoracic outlet syndrome or cervical spine problem. In some cases the radial pulse may be obliterated by the Adson maneuver, in which the chin is pointed up and turned to the involved side. This is a good indication of a scalenus anticus or cervical rib compression syndrome, which requires referral to a vascular surgeon. If the problem appears to arise in the cervical spine, the patient should be referred to a neurosurgeon. A soft, padded neck collar may provide temporary relief in either instance.

REFERENCES

1. Smith, J. R., and Graham, W. P., III: Nerves. *In* Kilgore, E. S., Jr., and Graham, W. P., III (eds).: The Hand: Surgical and Non-Surgical Management. Philadelphia, Lea & Febiger, 1977, pp. 211–248.

2. Spinner, M.: Injuries to the Major Branches of Peripheral Nerves of the Forearm. Philadelphia, W. B. Saunders, 1972.

15

Nontraumatic and Quasitraumatic Hand Problems

THE greater part of this book has been directed to the diagnosis and expeditious treatment or disposition of patients with acute traumatic hand problems. These are the problems most commonly encountered at a primary care level, especially in emergency departments. There remains a significant number of patients with nontraumatic or quasitraumatic problems of the hand who come to the physician's office or emergency department seeking a diagnosis and advice about treatment. Some of these problems have been discussed in prior chapters. In this chapter I briefly discuss arthritides of the hand, common hand tumors, and Dupuytren's disease. The discussions center on proper diagnosis and what reasonable advice these patients can be given. Some conservative measures to relieve acute discomfort are suggested.

Arthritides of the Hand

Arthritis or inflammation of joints falls into two broad categories. One is primarily a destructive proliferation of synovial tissue. Rheumatoid arthritis accounts for most of this type of arthritis, and any structure lined with synovium may become involved in this process—hence the common problems encountered with nerves and tendons as they go through synovial canals. The other type of arthritis involves destruction of the cartilaginous opposing surfaces of two articulating bones, often with hypertrophy of marginal bone. The prototype of this kind of arthritis is osteoarthritis or degenerative arthritis. Trauma may result in problems that combine features of each type of arthritis.

RHEUMATOID ARTHRITIS

This disease is a major crippler, not only of hands but of many other parts of the body. It may follow one of three clinical courses. A patient may have one attack with inflamed, tender joints that subsides and never recurs, leaving the patient with little or no residual disability. In a second type, the patient may have intermittent painful attacks that do not lead to a progressive degeneration of joints. Finally, a patient may have a steadily progressive form of the disease that destroys joints, disrupts tendons and leaves the hand ravaged as shown in Figures 15-1 and 15-2.

The early management of rheumatoid arthritis is medical, and moderation is the key word: moderate rest, moderate exercise, moderate diet, and avoidance of stress. Despite the appearance of many new anti-inflammatory drugs, aspirin remains the cornerstone of therapeutic medication. Although surgery may eventually be useful, primary referral of the patient should be to a rheumatologist or an internist with an interest in rheumatology.

In the hand the disease attacks the dorsal synovial extensor compartment, and proliferative synovitis may result (Fig. 15-3). Rupture of the extensor tendons often follows, which provides a good reason to refer the patient early for consideration for dorsal synovectomy. The entire wrist complex of joints may be totally destroyed by the process. The synovium in the carpal tunnel may proliferate to choke the median nerve and cause a carpal tunnel syndrome. The treatment suggested for this in Chapter 14 (injection of cortisone and splinting) may offer temporary relief, but usually surgical release and synovectomy are needed eventually.

Of the small finger joints, the MCPs are affected most seriously. Subluxation of the MCP joints with severe ulnar drift of the

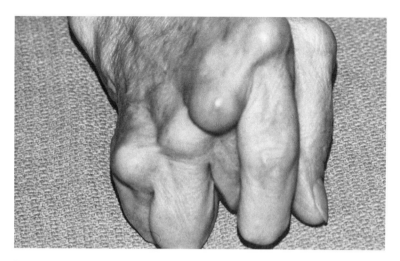

FIG. 15-1. *This elderly woman has advanced rheumatoid arthritis in her hands. The second through fifth MCP joints are dislocated and these digits have drifted ulnarly. She had difficulty opening her hands enough to grasp objects.*

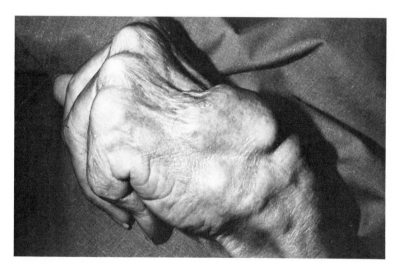

FIG 15-2. *This elderly man has some MCP subluxation and severe dorsal synovitis.*

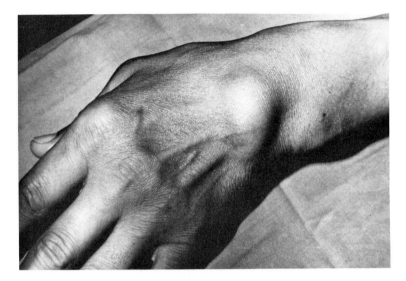

FIG 15-3. *A young adult patient with early dorsal synovitis as a manifestation of rheumatoid arthritis. The mass is softer and more diffuse than a ganglion; it moves proximally and distally as the MCP joints are flexed and extended.*

fingers is common (see Fig. 15-1). If a patient is seen at this stage of the disease for the first time, early referral to a hand surgeon is indicated. The earliest roentgenographic signs of MCP joint deterioration are periarticular erosions of the distal metacarpals. There is much debate about whether or not synovectomy performed at this early stage is helpful.

Although PIP joints are less frequently involved than MCP joints, they may be just as severely affected by the rheumatoid process with the development of either boutonniere or swan-neck deformities. In early stages, proliferation of the synovium may be quite painful.

Thumb deformities in rheumatoid arthritis may be either of the MCP flexion and IP extension type (which is more common), or the MCP extension and IP flexion type. Surgery often can help to correct these deformities, but it is not always successful.

Synovitis may overwhelm flexor tendon sheaths, and flexor tendon rupture may occur. Surgical synovectomy offers relief. DIP joints are relatively spared in many cases of rheumatoid arthritis.

Flexible implant arthroplasties of the Swanson or Niebauer type, or total joint replacement with prostheses of the Steffi type or others may offer the patient relief of deformity and improvement in function. However, none of these are panaceas, and it is unfair to promise a patient a surgical cure when in fact one is dealing with an often unremitting disease, and the best efforts of both internist and surgeon may offer only limited improvement.

DEGENERATIVE ARTHRITIS OR OSTEOARTHRITIS

This type of arthritis is quite common. In contrast to rheumatoid arthritis, which may occur at any age, this problem is confined to people in their forties and older. Degenerative arthritis most commonly affects the thumb basal joint (trapezial-first metacarpal) and the DIP joints.

Basal joint arthritis is a distressing problem because the thumb is used in a wide variety of ways in almost every hand function. Pain that occurs with compression activities (e.g., opening a pushbutton car door) is usually the earliest symptom, and it may be annoying or even disabling. The roentgenogram shows narrowing of the joint, sometimes with spur formation and ultimately partial subluxation.

Early treatment includes the administration of aspirin or other anti-inflammatory drugs, injection of intra-articular cortisone (in combination with lidocaine), and splinting. As the problem progresses, the thumb may assume an adducted stance and have greater pain and interference in function.

For progressive basal joint arthritis, a wide variety of surgical procedures have been used. These include fusion of the basal joint; removal of the trapezium and packing the space with autogenous material such as a tendon; Silastic wafer interposition; and total replacement of the trapezium with a Silastic prosthesis. (I favor the last method because trapezial articulations other than that with the first metacarpal may be involved.) In the primary care setting, one might explain these various possibilities to the patient, but not commit the consultant to an impossible course of action.

DIP joint involvement is common; it is the cause of "knobby knuckles" or Heberden's nodes so often seen in older patients. The roentgenogram (Fig. 15-4) shows joint narrowing and bony hypertrophy. Conservative treatment is administration of anti-inflammatory medication. Although other surgical treatments have been proposed, DIP fusion is the most practical procedure for unremitting symptoms. A fused DIP joint is cosmetically acceptable and causes few problems functionally.

A problem that is generally a consequence of DIP degenerative arthritis is the mucous cyst or ganglion of the DIP joint (Fig. 15-5). This ganglion is a cystic lesion that arises from the joint and may retain an open stalk to the joint; because of this conduit, it may wax and wane in size. Upon incision or spontaneous rupture, the typical clear, thick material of a ganglion is released. The connection with the joint can be demonstrated just prior to surgery by volar injection of the DIP joint with a dilute solution of methylene blue. The only practical treatment is surgical excision. The cyst must be traced to the DIP joint, where a bony spur will often be found. Sometimes a small skin graft is needed for wound closure.

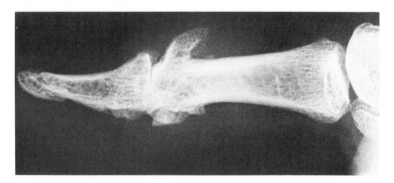

FIG. 15-4. *Roentgenogram of the thumb of a man in his middle sixties, showing advanced osteoarthritis with joint narrowing and striking osteophyte formation.*

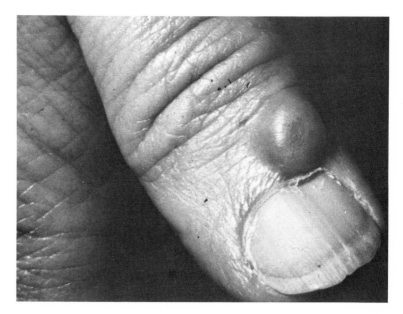

FIG. 15-5. *A typical and rather large mucous cyst.*

Surgery is often accompanied by an arthritic flare, and both patient and surgeon should be aware of this.

TRAUMATIC ARTHRITIS

Any joint subjected to trauma may develop chronic arthritis, which may resemble either the "wet" synovial proliferative arthritis or the "dry" degenerative osteoarthritis. Treatment must be individualized on the basis of the history and findings.

OTHER ARTHRITIDES

These include arthritis that results as a consequence of such conditions as psoriasis, the various so-called collagen diseases, Reiter's syndrome, and gonococcal infection (see Chapter 8). They are rarely encountered in everyday practice.

Hand Tumors

Except for warts and ganglions, hand tumors are uncommon or even rare. Treatment is usually surgical. The role of the primary care physician is diagnosis and referral in most instances.

WARTS

These horny dermal growths are probably viral in origin and may be difficult to eradicate. Aside from folk treatments, medical treatments are legion and include cauterization, surgical excision, and freezing with liquid nitrogen. A simple method to initiate treatment is to apply a salicylic acid pad cut to fit the lesion. This results in softening of the wart, which may then be scraped away every week or so. Most patients with warts should be referred to a dermatologist.

GANGLIONS

Ganglions are synovial cysts and therefore exist only where synovial tissue is present. The ganglion of the DIP joint has already been discussed.

The most common location for a hand ganglion is the dorsal wrist, usually on the radial side (Fig. 15-6). The next most common is the radial volar wrist. Ganglions in both locations usually arise from the radioscaphoid joint. Both may wax and wane in size presumably owing to intermittent intra-articular decompression.

The easiest way to display a ganglion on the dorsal wrist is to have the patient flex the wrist completely. The ganglion is usually firm to hard and transilluminable with a pen light; it does not move with the digital extrinsic extensors.

The classic treatment for the dorsal ganglion is the "Bible treatment," or hitting it hard with a large book. This makes the ganglion go away by rupturing it, but usually only temporarily; it is not a recommended treatment. Aspiration is not much more successful. Careful surgical extirpation down to the joint of origin under regional or general anesthesia in an operating room is the treatment of choice (Fig. 15-7). Patients should be warned that

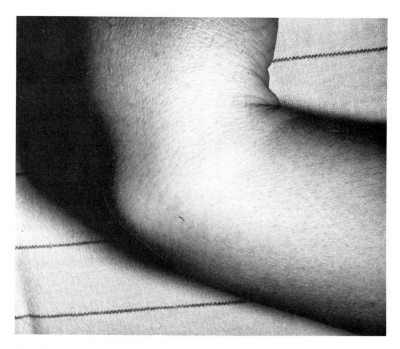

FIG. 15-6.   *Flexion of the wrist to display a ganglion.*

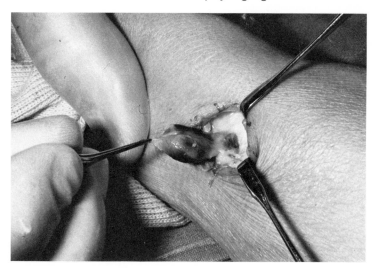

FIG. 15-7.   *Ganglionectomy is a formal operative procedure requiring the use of regional or general anesthesia and a tourniquet.*

they are trading a lump for a scar, and some may feel disinclined to surgery when that fact is explained.

Trauma, often trivial and forgotten, probably plays a role in the genesis of many ganglions. The trauma may be direct (a blow) or indirect (a twist of the wrist or forced flexion or extension). Ganglions may cause the patient actual discomfort with hand motion, concern about the significance of any unusual body mass, or concern over the cosmetic appearance. Splinting the wrist may provide temporary relief of pain for an acute ganglion.

Dorsal ganglions may be aspirated for diagnostic purposes; a viscid, clear fluid will be drawn into the syringe. Aspiration of a volar radial ganglion is not recommended because of the proximity of the radial artery. Anyone undertaking surgery of a radial volar ganglion should perform *and* record an Allen test (see p. 11).

Ganglions may occur at the volar finger base arising from the flexor tendon sheath. Often they occur after a blow or compression in this area. A ganglion in this area feels very hard and is a bit larger than a bee-bee. The recommended treatment is surgical removal with tourniquet control and local anesthesia in an operating room. Ganglions may also occur in the palm, but this location is far less frequent than the other three noted.

OTHER SOFT TISSUE TUMORS

The diagnosis of one of the uncommon tumors by a primary care physician may save the patient much trouble in getting a correct diagnosis and proper treatment. *Lipomas*, although common elsewhere in the body, are uncommon in the hand. Generally they are softer than ganglions and do not transmit light as do ganglions. *Inclusion cysts* are firm like ganglions, but they may be located anywhere. They follow trauma that causes an ingrowth of epithelial cells. *Giant cell tumors* may occur anywhere on the fingers or hand (usually volarly). The key to the correct diagnosis is their multilobulated appearance, which can be felt even through intact skin. At surgery they are yellow, multilobulated, and arise from connective tissue. Careful removal of *all* the tumor is necessary to prevent local recurrence, but these tumors do not metastasize. *Hemangiomas* may be small or large; generally they are soft and have a bluish cast. Surgery is the treatment of choice. *Glomus tumors* are growths of the neuromyoarterial apparatus, and they usually occur under the nail in the nailbed. The clue to their correct diagnosis is that they are intensely, exquisitely tender. This diagnosis is often missed, and if you make it correctly and refer the patient for surgical treatment, he or she will be grateful.

Pyogenic granuloma is a curious lesion that often alarms patients because of its rapid growth and frightening appearance (Fig. 15-8). It is an overgrowth of granulation tissue at the site of an injury. It is highly vascular and friable, and is treated by snipping it off at the base and controlling the hemorrhage with cautery. Occasionally deeper excision and formal closure are necessary.

Keratoacanthoma is a scaly, slightly raised lesion with a central keratin plug (Fig. 15-9). It spontaneously regresses, but because it looks so much like squamous cell carcinoma, the only way to establish a definite diagnosis is by histologic examination.

Seborrheic keratoses are brown spots that may dot the skin in older people; they look as if they are "stuck on." They may be left alone or removed by cryosurgery.

Nevi or moles may be *junctional, intradermal,* or *compound.* The former appear as flat macules ranging in color from brown to black. The latter two look more alike and appear heaped up on top of the skin. They have no malignant potential. Nevi may be left alone, except when they occur subungually. Any pigmented subungual lesion should be removed.

A *premalignant* soft tissue tumor is *actinic keratosis* or sun spot. These tumors are small, red, scaling spots induced by the cumulative effects of sunlight, radiation, or chemicals. They should be removed, usually by cryosurgery.

MALIGNANT SOFT TISSUE TUMORS

Basal cell carcinoma is a nodule that ulcerates centrally; it should be removed. *Squamous cell carcinoma* is a red ulcerating lesion that may metastasize. Twenty-five percent of actinic keratoses progress to this lesion. The deadliest of all the malignant

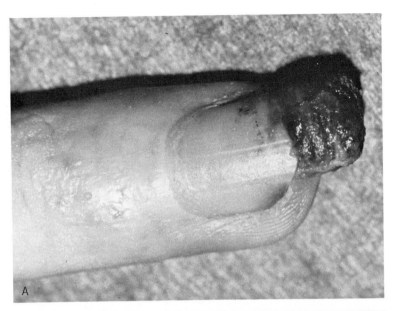

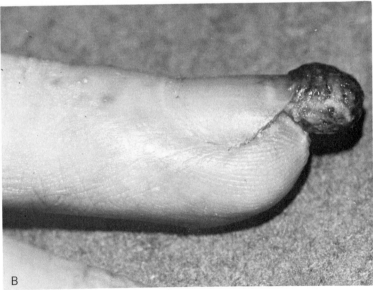

FIG. 15-8.   (A and B) Pyogenic granuloma.

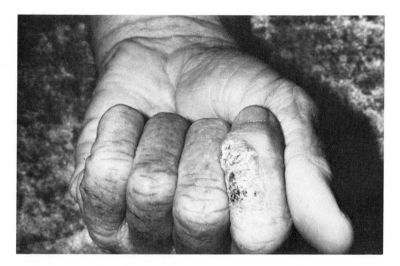

FIG. 15-9. *The only way to distinguish this keratoacanthoma from a squamous cell carcinoma is by histologic examination.*

tumors is *malignant melanoma.* These tumors are pigmented nodules, and any growth, change of color, or itchiness of a pigmented nodule may indicate the presence of this tumor. Hutchinson's sign of periungual pigmentation is an especially ominous sign for a subungual melanoma. About one fifth of malignant melanomas are amelanotic (i.e., unpigmented). Any lesion suspected of being a melanoma should be surgically excised and histologically identified.

BONY TUMORS

These are even more unusual than soft tissue tumors, with one exception: enchondroma (Fig. 15-10). This is often an incidental roentgenographic finding. It is not a malignant tumor, but will grow until the cortex becomes so thin that fracture occurs. Patients with this lesion should be referred for curettage of the lesion and packing with bone chips.

Other bony or joint tumors are rarely seen, and if the primary care physician encounters a case, the patient should be promptly referred to a specialist.

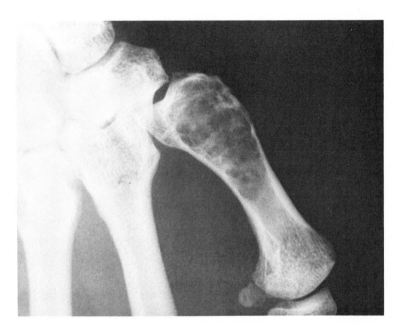

FiG. 15-10.   *A typical enchondroma.*

Dupuytren's Disease

This problem occurs mainly in white males in late middle age, but it may also affect women, young men, and black men. There are various theories about the cause of Dupuytren's disease and various diseases (alcoholism, diabetes) with which it is said to be associated. Although many patients want to attribute the problem to trauma, this has never been demonstrated as a cause.

The disease starts as a subcutaneous nodule, usually in the palm, and may progress along the vertical bands of the palmar fascia, causing skin dimpling and eventually contracture at the MCP, PIP, and rarely, DIP joints. The process does not involve the flexor tendons. As it advances, however, it becomes anchored to the metacarpals by the so-called vertical septae and the tendons are so surrounded (although surgically quite separate) that the uninitiated examiner may be fooled.

The typical picture of Dupuytren's contracture (Fig. 15-11) is unmistakable. When the disease is confined to a digit without palmar involvement, the clinical picture is also quite characteristic if you are aware of the pattern.

Early stages of the disease may be characterized by soreness and itching of the nodule, and relief but not cure is afforded with

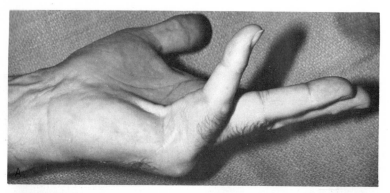

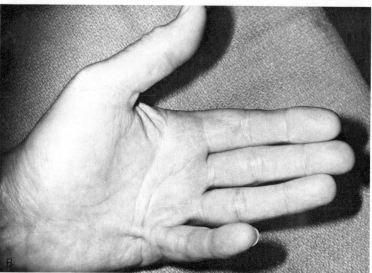

FIG. 15-11 *(A and B). Typical Dupuytren's fasciitis and contracture in the hand of a man in his late fifties.*

local injections of cortisone. It is impossible to predict either the chance or rate of progression.

Surgery should be confined to contractures that bother the patient. In my opinion this should consist of fasciectomy of the involved tissue, not fasciotomy. This is a purely elective procedure, but should not be undertaken by the unaware because of the close proximity to and intermeshing with the digital nerves. Refer the patient to a hand surgeon.

REFERENCES

1. Flatt, A. E.: The Care of the Rheumatoid Hand. 3rd ed. St. Louis, C. V. Mosby, 1974.

2. Cooley, S. G. E.: Tumors of the hand and forearm. *In* Converse, J. M., and McCarthy, J. G. (eds.): Reconstructive Plastic Surgery. (Vol. 6, The Hand and Upper Extremity, ed. by J. W. Littler) Philadelphia, W. B. Saunders, 1977.

3. Boyes, J. H.: Dupuytren's contracture. *In* Bunnell's Surgery of the Hand. 5th ed. Philadelphia, J. B. Lippincott, 1970, pp. 225–239.

Index

269